CANDLING
for Optimal Health

Common and Lesser Known Benefits

A Seeker's Guide to a Life Worth Living
Les bougies auriculaires et leurs bienfaits méconnus (in French)
Messages from Beyond the Veil

CANDLING
for Optimal Health

Common and Lesser Known Benefits

JILI HAMILTON

 FINDHORN PRESS

The right of Jili Hamilton to be identified as the author
of this work has been asserted by her in accordance
with the Copyright, Designs and Patents Act 1998.

First edition published by Pen Press Publishers, England
Revised edition published in 2014 by Findhorn Press, Scotland

ISBN 978-1-84409-130-0

A CIP record for this title is available from the British Library.

Edited by Nicky Leach
Cover design by Richard Crookes
Interior design by Damian Keenan
Printed and bound in the EU

Published by
Findhorn Press
117-121 High Street,
Forres IV36 1AB,
Scotland, UK

t +44 (0)1309 690582
f +44 (0)131 777 2711
e info@findhornpress.com
www.findhornpress.com

Contents

Disclaimer

EAR CANDLING is not considered to be a medical treatment, and no claim of this nature is made. Always read and follow the directions provided with ear candles, or seek guidance from an experienced ear candle practitioner. All information contained in this book is intended to increase knowledge of candling, its origins, and uses, but it is not a substitute for medical advice or treatment for specific medical conditions.

The information is given in good faith and is neither intended to diagnose any physical or mental condition nor to serve as a substitute for informed medical advice or care. Please contact your health professional for medical advice and treatment. Neither author nor publisher can be held liable by any person for any loss or damage whatsoever that may arise from the use of this book or any of the information therein.

Acknowledgments

Many people have helped me in the preparation of the various editions of my book on ear candles. Vicky Lee, my dentist in London, gave me the initial push to start setting down on paper my knowledge and experience of the subject. Before that, Lisha Simester, as part of the organizing team of the Healing Arts Exhibition in London in 1991, provided me with the opportunity I needed to start exhibiting and demonstrating the candles.

Deep gratitude is also due to Patrick Quanten, MD and Greg Webb, RMT, who have not only given me permission to use their very informative paper on the use of candles in the treatment of cancer but whose wide experience and generosity have enabled me to add some fascinating new material in this updated version. Patrick, in particular, with his profound knowledge, has always been ready to answer my questions and has thereby added volumes to my understanding of candling.

Joy Picot gave me some excellent examples of successful treatments. She was kind enough to check that the details were right, and I'm extremely grateful to her. Cynthia Burren also gave me a fascinating piece of information.

Wendy Rigby supported me at many exhibitions, and her professional advice as a teacher and therapist was just what I needed at that time.

My thanks, too, to Emmanuel Berrod for his photography and to my patient models.

Last, but by no means least, my heartfelt gratitude to all my patients and students, who have taught me (and are continuing to teach me) so much.

Author's Note

This book is a follow-up to my previous publication *Hopi Candles*, and I have retained the basic information and some of the examples that appeared in the first book. At the time the last edition was published, in 2006, I felt I had said everything I had to say about ear candles and ear problems. How wrong I was! This time I won't risk making a prediction, as I have learnt a lot more, uncovered a great deal of new material, and, as a result, the content of this new edition has more than doubled.

An International Ear Candling Conference, at which I was privileged to present a session, was held in England in November 2006. There, I discovered more examples of successful candling and some amazing new ways in which the candles have proved their efficacy. (See Chapter 6.)

My aim has always been to inform the general public as well as other practitioners of what the candles can do and what conditions can be treated. To this end, fact sheets relating to how candles work on children, female problems, hearing loss, sinusitis, stress, the immune system and tinnitus can be downloaded from my website: *www.jilihamilton.com.*

Candling is by no means the only way to treat certain health issues, and there is plenty of information out there on other effective therapies. Ear candles can be a very useful addition to whatever therapeutic approach you choose and can lead to an even better result, so don't rule out combining therapies. In this book, I cover alternative solutions and have tried to give as much information as possible on vaccines and ototoxic medication without boring the lay reader by being too detailed or too technical.

Every aspect of a patient's lifestyle is important. For example, if someone is receiving treatment for sinus problems but continues to eat quantities of dairy produce, then there will be little progress; the candles will help initially, but the effect won't be lasting. This is due to the fact that cow's milk in particular can increase the mucus in the system and that's not helpful for someone with blocked sinuses. It is always important to take a holistic approach and, as I hope to demonstrate in this book, as the candles stimulate the immune system, everyone can benefit in some way.

I am an enthusiastic networker and am always happy to hear from readers with queries or information. I can be contacted at *info@jilihamilton.com*, or alternatively, I welcome visits to my website: *www.jilihamilton.com*.

Introduction

It was whilst living in Switzerland in the late 1980s that I first heard the word 'reflexology'. A friend showed me a diagram of the reflex zones on the feet and how, by stimulating the appropriate zone, the corresponding organ in the body could be treated. This was so fascinating that I decided to look into it further, and I qualified as a reflexologist in 1988.

It was the start of a passion for complementary medicine; in fact, it was just after obtaining my diploma that my attention was caught by an article in a magazine about ear treatment candles. It was accompanied by a photograph of a man lying on one side with a hand holding a lighted taper upright in his ear. Very bizarre! However, on reading the article, I learnt that these candles (which are hollow tubes made from linen or cotton and not exactly 'candles' as we know them) could be used for a multitude of health problems. Ear cones are just as popular and have exactly the same function, and many people prefer to use them. **NOTE:** For simplicity I've used the word 'candle' throughout the text but the word 'cone' may easily be substituted.

The treatment seemed extremely basic, consisting of lighting this tube, said to work for sinusitis, otitis, impacted wax, relaxation and so on, and placing it over the entrance to the auditory canal. This enabled the flow of energy to the ear to be improved through stimulation of the acupressure points and the lymphatic system. The article added that once these systems functioned properly, the production of wax was controlled and the energy flow normalized.

A couple of days later, I was contacted on another matter by someone I'd met on my reflexology course. I mentioned candling to her and she became very enthusiastic, telling me she had used ear candles for years and then recounted a few cases where she had found them hugely effective. Convinced that I too wanted to try candling, I wrote down the name of a lady who made them, then a friend, who was as interested in the technique as I was, visited her and purchased some candles. I received my first treatment and before long was treating my work colleagues and obtaining excellent results.

When I moved to London from Switzerland, in 1989, I was amazed to find that candling was not widely known in the UK and decided to set up a company to import and promote the candles. Our first public demonstration took place at the Healing Arts Exhibition in London in the autumn of 1991. This is the oldest and largest exhibition of complementary therapies in the UK and attracts hundreds of exhibitors and thousands of visitors from all over the world. From Day 1, we were caught up in an amazing rush of enthusiasm, with people practically standing on each other's shoulders to obtain a better view! Some of the visitors told me that they made their own ear candles with more or less success, so they were delighted to find something being produced commercially that was safe.

Sales of ear candles soared and included many repeat orders. I was frequently contacted by people who had marvellous stories to tell and, perhaps more importantly, by people who couldn't find any information on the candles. Indeed, although more information is now available, for most of the time I have been using ear candles, I have found practically no published information—apart from a few magazine articles and plenty of ill-informed comments on how dangerous or what a waste of space they are.

For example, it has often puzzled me how people can say that a candle treatment is painful because, when done properly, it is wonderfully relaxing. Recently, I trained two therapists, one of whom already knows the candles and treats her family when she visits them. She couldn't understand why she was unable to feel the candle and insisted it was not in place. If this is the case, smoke will emanate from the base. Now I understand that people who do not know how to do a treatment think they should 'screw' the candle into the auditory canal (the outer ear), but this can be excruciatingly painful. I also understand why smaller ear candles for children are sold, although they are totally unnecessary.

When the candle is placed *lightly over the entrance to the auditory canal* the size of the ear has no importance whatsoever. It made me even more convinced that a book on ear candling is absolutely essential for people who want to candle and even more so for people receiving paying patients. After all, you don't want to spend good money to writhe in agony on a therapist's table!

My original intention in writing this book, putting into it what I have learnt and am still learning about ear candles and what they can do, still stands, and this edition vastly expands the content of what has gone before. If it helps to introduce more people to this simple but highly effective therapy, if it helps more people to learn how to do a treatment properly, then I shall feel it has been totally worthwhile.

Over the years I have been using them, I can say with conviction that ear candles do everything they are advertised as doing, and much more. Candling has often been considered something anyone could perform at home, and ear candles have always been on sale in pharmacies and health food shops. However, from what I've learnt since first writing this Introduction, I'm positive that, although using the candles at home is an excellent idea—especially for children, for relaxation, or for a rapid result—the moment a more serious health problem arises, your best option is to consult a therapist who can look at a particular pathology holistically. This is especially true in the case of long-standing conditions that may have proved difficult to treat by other means. Some professional therapists who use ear candles combine them with different therapies, as I do myself. It is worth emphasizing that all forms of complementary medicine go hand in hand with a healthy lifestyle; this applies to every aspect of our lives, not just to our nutritional habits.

When we have a health problem it fills our waking hours, but when it disappears we immediately forget about it. I have discovered that when receiving patients for a follow-up treatment they often tell me that nothing has changed. Perhaps the problem on which they had focused hasn't improved, but when I question them more closely

I find that, well, yes, they have slept better; well, yes, they have had more regular bowel movements; well, yes, they did have a runny nose for 24 hours and then the congestion disappeared, and so on. This is why I recommend consulting a properly trained therapist for a long-standing or intractable problem, so that, together, patient and therapist can measure progress.

I do want to reiterate that for those conditions that have suddenly arisen, such as the onset of a cold, blocked sinuses, a child with earache, a stressful day at work, the candles can be a wonderful panacea. They are, however, a *complementary* therapy; they do not replace proper medical care. It is important to remember this, and act accordingly.

CHAPTER 1

History and Use of Candling

Many people who visited our stand at health exhibitions in the early days expressed amazement at seeing a treatment that to them was something granny did when they were children. I have met people from Australasia, all round the Mediterranean basin, Asia and the Americas, as well as many other places, who say that this was a well-known folk remedy in their home country and they are delighted to see it again.

One therapist from Cyprus told me that people in his village used paper impregnated with beeswax and honey to make cones, and it is a therapy much in use even today. As I didn't at the time know why honey was used, his mother was able to tell me that it stopped the cone from burning down too fast. Rolled-up newspaper or tobacco leaves have also been mentioned many times. Each country's traditional method grew out of its most easily obtainable materials. Pottery cones and even reusable glass cones have also turned up.

Whether candles or cones, everyone seems to agree that candling is a very ancient tradition, stretching back for centuries, to the time when folk healers all over the world used the therapy in some form or another. Chinese, Tibetan, Egyptian, Mayan, Aztec, and several North American Indian cultures are invariably mentioned as performing candling ceremonies. Traditionally, the Choctaw Indians of the south-eastern United States have used a method that involves blowing the smoke from various herbs through a cone-shaped object into the ear canal, while shamans in the Muskogee tribe of Oklahoma rolled the leaves that grow around corn cobs to use in shamanic

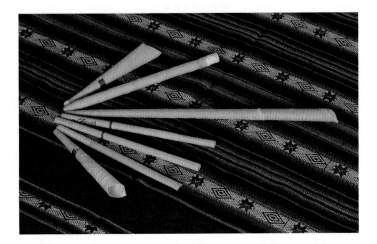

candling rituals. In Italy, people used cheese cloth; in India, they used dried-out papyrus seeds for candling.

Many ancient cultures thought of coning as a spiritual practice to clear the mind and the senses, as the pathologies that cause us problems today were largely unknown to our ancestors. Using the ear candles to improve health, therefore, would not have been a consideration. I feel that, even after all these years, we have merely scratched the surface of the many uses for candles.

Today's Methods

Let me say first of all that ear candles are *not* used for cleaning the ears, as most people seem to think. Our ears (and our auditory system) are constructed in such a way that they work perfectly without any 'help' from us. However, with dietary lapses, stress, medication, and so forth, our bodies don't always function as well as they should. The energies circulate more sluggishly, and people can find that their ears seem 'blocked'. By far the most widespread method of dealing with this is syringing, a process performed in a doctor's surgery whereby a high-pressure jet of water is released into the ear aimed at dislodging and extracting hardened wax—and extremely unpleasant it can be, too, depending on the expertise of the practitioner. Apart from the possibility of perforating the eardrum (rare, but it has been known to occur), people find the more they have it done the more they need it done. The stimulus to the ear is unnatural and very powerful, and the cleansing is perhaps too thorough, causing the body to produce more wax to compensate. This is why people who decide to try the candles to clear blockages will need more than one treatment—it is gentle, and the amount of wax that needs to come to the surface does so only when it is ready. A normal, healthy amount of ear wax is replaced in 24–48 hours, and when the energies are circulating properly the ears don't get blocked.

This is just one well-known use for the ear candles, but it isn't one of the major reasons why people resort to candling. Indeed, those who consult me are suffering from a wide variety of health problems—problems that would not necessarily lead us to think of ear candles as the first line of approach. They have possibly read articles or seen or heard interviews I have given; some have read earlier versions of my book and have learnt that the candles have been used successfully for many different pathologies.

When it comes to treating a patient with a long-standing and/ or difficult health problem, a trained ear candling therapist is the best person to advise on the suggested number of treatments to resolve the condition; s/he may also refer the patient to other health professionals, trained in nutritional therapy, cranial osteopathy, and other complementary therapies, as s/he deems necessary. Qualified ear candling practitioners can be found in several countries. They are graduates of professional courses in ear candling (or ototherapy, as it is called in Switzerland) who have obtained a recognized qualification—something that many patients find reassuring (see Candling Courses at the back of this book). The people I have trained all practise other therapies. A first candling consultation should include questions on your lifestyle and basic information on what to avoid and what to do. For example, if you drink 10 coffees a day and one glass of water, the therapist would point out that the reverse is likely to be a better option.

The candles we use in Europe are either thin, hollow linen tubes or cones of varying lengths and sizes impregnated with wax, honey,

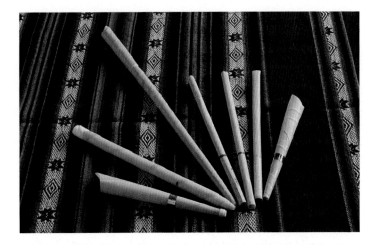

herbs, and/or essential oils. People often ask if they will be burnt by hot wax. Based on my experience, I can tell you unequivocally that that won't happen with properly produced candles. First, only a small amount of wax is used in the manufacture and, second, the linen or cotton burns like any other material and the candle is designed not to drip or break. **NOTE:** ear candles with a filter are made in such a way that nothing can 'fall down' the candle and burn the recipient and are infinitely preferable.

If you open the stub of the ear candle left after the treatment, you will find that any residue is lodged between the filter and the burnt part, never, ever between the filter and the ear. This residue comes from the candle, obviously not from the patient's ear, and is a way of refuting any suggestion that the candle draws wax out of the ear; it does nothing of the sort. You will see a little powder residue in the ear after the treatment, but this should be left alone: it will make its own way out.

Whichever brand of ear candle you use, it is *essential* to read, understand, and follow the instructions. I have prepared a very clear instruction sheet, which I give to everyone who purchases candles from me for home use.

Whichever make you choose, do buy properly produced candles made from pure, top-quality, *natural* ingredients. Candles with an

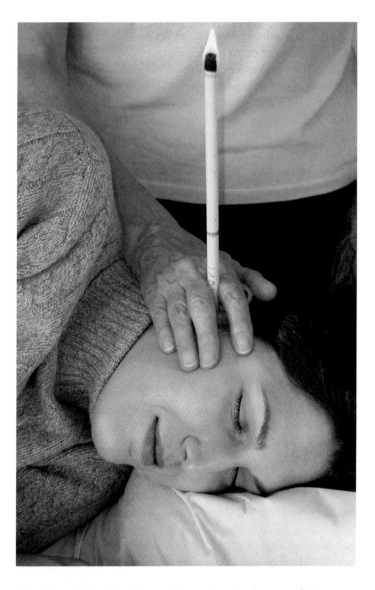

aluminium lining should never be used, as the dangers of this material (especially when heated) are well known and have been linked to
Alzheimer's disease.

It is also important to avoid candles made from paraffin wax as this by-product of petrol, sometimes used to rigidify the ear candle, is highly toxic and can cause irritation. The same can be said for candles made from soy, which is invariably genetically modified (GM). Candles made from organic cotton or linen will be beige or yellowish; those that are pure white are unlikely to be made from natural materials and are either synthetic or cotton bleached with chemicals. As with anything else, candles made from organic materials are bound to have a higher vibration.

How the Candles Work

If we take the view (which quantum physicists now seem to have proved beyond any doubt) that everything is energy, the body is no exception. When the body's energy is circulating properly we are healthy and positive. However, most of us eat food that may have been treated with chemicals and is often full of sugar, salt, and poor-quality fats from processed or junk foods, including vegetable oils such as corn oil, which are too high in omega 6 fatty acids; in addition, we live in polluted environments and lead stressful lives. All of these factors help to lower our resistance and then we fall ill.

One of the primary functions of ear candles is to stimulate the body's energy, which they do very powerfully and effectively. This is why some people who have used candles for one problem, such as migraine, have found to their delight that their sinuses clear, too. Or those who have used them for sinusitis have found their hearing improves at the same time.

The greatest advantage of the candles, therefore, is that they work on the immune system. Debris is carried along a network of capillaries by a fluid called lymph, and it is purified through the lymphatic ganglions, which are found all over the body; when lymph is flowing as it should, it prevents us from falling ill. It circulates through these capillaries in the same manner as blood circulates through the veins, but as the lymphatic system has no pumping mechanism to allow it to circulate, it relies on the movement of muscles to create peristalsis that pushes it around. The whole body receives a boost from candling, which, because it enhances energy naturally, affects the functioning of the lymphatic system (you will find more information on this in Chapter 4). This is also why candles can be so effective for constipated patients as, once the lymph is doing its job properly and removing waste products to be filtered and excreted, patients invariably find themselves having more frequent and easier bowel movements.

Acupressure points, which are found everywhere on the body, are also stimulated in the region of the ear by the candle treatment. If we take the shape of the ear as an inverted foetus (and it was Paul Nogier who discovered this fact in the 1950s), we can find to which zones these acupressure points relate. It is said that pirates had pierced ear-lobes because, representing the eye reflex, this enabled them to see ships coming over the horizon before the ships' lookouts saw them! It is also a fact that people who have piercings elsewhere on the ear can suffer from certain zones being overstimulated.

An extremely detailed explanation of the way the candles work is given in a paper entitled *Ear Candling and Cancer Therapy* by Patrick Quanten, MD (UK) and Greg Webb, RMT (Canada), which, with the authors' permission, I have reproduced in its entirety in Chapter 5, so I won't repeat the information here.

A crystal therapist, watching a treatment being given at an exhibition, claimed that she could see negativity being burned out of the aura (the electromagnetic field surrounding the body), and this is one of the more subtle functions of the candle. It is why it needs to be held upright and why getting up too quickly after a treatment can cause a feeling of light-headedness. One of the students on my professional course remarked that for him the act of burning a candle opened the door between the two worlds, and this does fit with what the crystal therapist was seeing.

It is extremely important to rest for 10–15 minutes once the burning has stopped to enable the effect of the treatment to circulate throughout the system. This also happens when we receive a massage or any other complementary therapy: what the therapist has done is to stimulate the energy, and we derive far more benefit from it if we can take things easy for a while afterwards. Therapists understand energy and how it works, but unless someone using the candles un-

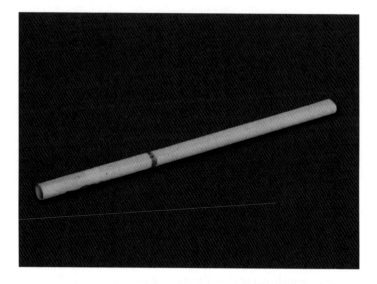

derstands this, he or she will not really be able to get to grips with the finer points of the treatment. Of course, the physical result will be there, but understanding how energy works opens us up to a whole new way of looking at ear candles.

This leads me to say that the act of candling is the *start* of a process to get the energies circulating. A positive result does not necessarily happen during the treatment, and the patient may even feel less well afterwards; s/he will have a better idea of the benefits of the treatment after a good night's sleep, or even after another treatment. It is important to bear in mind that the longer someone has been suffering from a particular complaint the longer it may take to get to the root cause. As we are all different, it is never possible to say just how long, but as a general guideline I recommend three treatments over a period of 4–6 weeks to see if the candles can be beneficial for a patient. If they can (and although it may not seem to be so, a worsening of the pathology is actually a *positive* indicator), further treatments are definitely advisable. If the candles don't appear to be making a difference, then an alternative therapy should be tried, although it should be pointed out that even if the initial problem doesn't seem to have responded, the body has found a more pressing need elsewhere for the energy generated by the candle. Energy flows to where it is most needed, so there will always be some benefit.

Why would a worsening of the condition be considered a good result? With complementary therapies, healing starts from the inside, whereas allopathic medicine is geared toward removing the symptoms and not addressing the root cause. I had a rather frustrating case of a young woman who had taken several courses of antibiotics and wanted to try natural healing methods. She enjoyed the treatment and was booked to return in two weeks. However, although I *always* explain that complementary therapies take time to work for long-standing problems, that things can get worse before they get better, and gave her an information sheet—something I hand out to every new patient—the act of candling brought out a latent infection. She immediately consulted an allopathic practitioner who gave her antibiotics, and she cancelled her next appointment, telling me she might try again when she had recovered!

The worsening of a condition is a call to listen to what the body is telling us. Nothing, I repeat, nothing is 'caused' through using the candles. There are certain contraindications to treatment, which are described more fully later on: for example, if a patient already has eczema or dryness in the outer ear, the warmth of the candle will dry this out further and cause irritation and discomfort. If, however, someone has an infection that is lying dormant, perhaps already having been treated with allopathic medicine, the symptoms may have gone but the root cause has not been addressed, so the act of candling could well bring it to the surface, which is what probably happened in the case mentioned above. It is certainly not a commentary on 'what the candles did' but a valuable message to listen to what our bodies are trying to tell us.

When the only physical action of the candles is to sit lightly over the entrance to the auditory canal and send warm energy downwards, it is evident that they can't, in and of themselves, cause illness. The energy circulated by the action of the candles can never do any harm, either: it goes right to the spot where the patient needs it most, and even if s/he decides that the candles have had little effect on the initial problem, it could be that the energy systems of other regions of the body have a higher priority and, once these have been dealt with, the whole system will start to function at a higher frequency. That is where it is essential for a therapist to question the patient when s/he returns because, as I have already mentioned, so many general improvements may have occurred without the patient making the connection with the candles or even noticing their effect.

When people come for a treatment, I advise them against washing their hair the same day or using a mobile phone or an iPod, and in cold weather to bring a scarf or hat to cover their ears on the way home. I received one new patient at a health centre, and when I gave her this information she announced that she already had plans to go to the swimming pool for a swim straight afterwards! This is a contraindication, but it might not be evident to someone who is unaware of how the candles work. Another patient told me she had slept with ear plugs for many years (even when she goes away somewhere quiet) and could no longer sleep without them. She admitted she often had to have her ears syringed to get rid of the build-up of wax. The candles cannot offer much in this case, as our body's intelligence is awesome and complete and no bodily orifice, each having its own particular function, should ever be blocked up systematically and for no good reason. Our cells and our autonomic nervous system never take a break, and essential work is being carried out while we sleep.

As mentioned earlier, there is a lot of disinformation around. For example, my attention was drawn to an article by an ear, nose, and throat practitioner who expressed the view that the candles were useless and dangerous as he had seen a whole catalogue of 'adverse' effects. At least one of these 'adverse' effects was physically impossible, and as for the rest: either the candle had exploded or the person treating was holding it lighted side down! I have given thousands of treatments over a quarter of a century, and the only 'adverse' effect I have experienced is when candling has set off a healing crisis and the stimulation to the immune system has awakened a latent infection in the body. (See above and also the entry for Sinusitis in Chapter 2.) I am sure that if he *had* seen such problems after candling (which I doubt), they had all come from the same source.

Benefits of Using the Candles

The following are among the many physical conditions for which ear candles have proved beneficial. I have more information about some cases than I do about others, but I wanted to share what I have learnt. We are not all alike, and treatments that have been successful for one or two patients may not give the same result in someone else. It could also be that one patient will require many more treatments than another. However, as the candles can never do any harm, if the patient is agreeable, I'm always prepared to try using them for something not yet in their repertoire (or mine). Indeed, this is how I have made so many fascinating discoveries, including the effective use of candling for:

- Age-related deafness
- Cancer
- Candida
- Constipation and haemorrhoids
- Excessive wax
- Flying (discomfort when the cabin pressure drops before landing)
- Glaucoma
- Glue ear
- Hay fever and other allergies
- Hearing problems
- Mastoid discomfort
- Migraines and headaches
- Painful periods
- Relaxation
- Sinus problems
- Skin disorders
- Sleep apnoea
- Stress relief
- Swimming and diving (water lodging in the ear)
- Tinnitus
- Vertigo and Ménière's Disease

and there are certainly many more (see Chapters 2, 6, and 7).

What Constitutes a Treatment?

All that is needed is a pair of ear candles or cones, a small bowl of water, a lighter or matches and some lavender-scented cream or essential oil. If the manufacturer recommends anything else, such as scissors, ensure that you have these to hand, too. The person administering the treatment must have read and understood the instructions and must not be working in a draught. I use a purpose-made cloth to protect the hair and face. Why? Because it looks more professional and the patient feels more reassured.

I like to start a treatment by massaging the patient's legs and feet or head to promote relaxation and to open the body's energy, although it is important to ensure that they are comfortable with this idea. Some people do not like the idea of their feet being touched or their head being massaged, so it is essential to consult them; if they demur, I skip this part of the procedure. I have had patients with verrucas and eczema on their feet, so it goes without saying that I would not massage them.

I then ask the patient if s/he has an ear or side of the body that functions better. The treatment starts with the patient lying on the 'weaker' side. The reason for beginning with the 'best' ear is that once the first side has been treated, the localized energy circulation has been improved, making it easier to treat the other, weaker side. It's like an exam where we look at all the questions on the paper and work on the easy ones first to put us in the mood for tackling the more difficult ones.

One golden rule is that candling must always be carried out on both ears and the candle must burn down to the same level each side. This is because our balance mechanism is located in the inner ear and the two sides need to receive an equal amount of treatment. It is also why it is possible, when working on small children, either to use a cone, which is normally shorter, or to stop burning a candle well before the mark. (See also Chapter 2: Children and Candles.)

Once the patient is comfortably settled (covered by a light blanket and with a small pillow supporting the head), the candle is lit at the appropriate end and placed gently over the entrance to the auditory canal. To do this, pull *very lightly* on the outside of the ear to give a clearer view of where to place the candle. When it's correctly positioned, the patient should hardly notice its presence. First-time users often ask: 'Is it in place? I can't feel it'. It will immediately be evident if it is not because smoke will emanate from the base. If this happens, *slightly* change the position of the candle and waft the smoke carefully away with your free hand, but if it means the candle is no longer upright, then gently push the patient's chin down towards the pillow to get the correct angle. For someone who is candling for the first time it can be helpful to ask the patient to insert the candle, as s/he will know exactly where it should sit. During the treatment the patient is often aware of a crackling sound—it is very comforting and has been likened to lying in front of a log fire.

The candle should be allowed to burn down to an inch or so from the end, where there may be a printed guide-mark. On reaching this point, or just above it, carefully remove the stub and extinguish it in the bowl of water. When using a cone, there is invariably a very clear mark; some brands are even self-extinguishing.

Once the treatment is complete, a little lavender-scented cream may be massaged behind and around each ear, and the patient must be kept warm and comfortable and encouraged to rest for at least 10 minutes. Here, the therapist can do a light face or foot massage, if the patient has agreed to it beforehand—I do 10–15 minutes of Reiki, during which time the patient invariably falls asleep.

A glass of water should be provided for the patient to drink when s/he sits up at the end of the treatment, as the act of swallowing opens up the Eustachian tubes. If the candling is being done at home, the best time to treat is just before going to bed. From feedback I have received, it seems that even if patients need to go out and drive home afterwards, they invariably have an excellent night's sleep.

Candling is a very gentle process and should be relaxing, so if you consult someone who causes any pain at all by pushing the candle too far in, either protest or get up and leave immediately. Ear candles are not dangerous, the therapy is not dangerous, but people practising it without a clear idea of how to do it can certainly be dangerous.

Getting the Best Out of the Treatment

When candling is done at home, people may feel that it is not necessary to re-create the calm atmosphere one would expect in a professional setting, although like anything else, the circumstances in which a treatment is given and received make a great difference to its efficacy. Appropriate music can be played but do check first, as this can cause an overload for the ears and I don't suggest it. It is important to ensure that there are no draughts in the room, as this would cause the candle to burn down too fast and blow the flame in all directions.

When I demonstrated candling on my stand at health exhibitions, there was always a lot of noise and much coming and going, so it was difficult to create optimum conditions. I did once experiment with someone who came two days in succession. On the first occasion, he was unimpressed with how he felt afterwards, likely because I was alone on the stand and talking to visitors at the same time as I was treating him. The next day my colleagues were with me, giving me a chance to concentrate on my patient (which would be the setting when working in a private therapy room or candling at home). He fell asleep on that occasion, clearly demonstrating that the conditions in which the therapy is carried out are as important as the action of the candle itself.

I suggest that the person giving the treatment places his or her hand *very lightly* over the ear with the candle sticking up between the fingers; this gives a feeling of reassurance to the patient and cuts him/her off from anything that is going on around. The ear can also be protected by the cloth I've mentioned earlier. If the person giving the treatment is a hands-on or Reiki healer, s/he will understand the benefit to the patient of having the hand gently placed over the ear and s/he will be able to channel healing energy at the same time. However, if the person giving the treatment is unsure, it's enough just to follow the instructions that come with the candles and the illustrations on the sheet. It is as well to ensure that the candle is properly in place before putting your hand over the ear, as you will not notice right away if smoke is emanating from the base and it will need a little more effort to clear it.

For people suffering from blocked sinuses, it is a good idea to put several drops each of peppermint and eucalyptus oils on a tissue and press it to any part of the body. The oils will be rapidly absorbed by the skin and travel through the bloodstream, thus enabling the patient to breathe more clearly after several minutes.

Multiple Treatments

As candling is quite powerful, no more than one pair of candles need be used at one time, although in an emergency the treatment could be repeated over several days. This will not only promote healing by purifying the lymph but will keep the passages clear so that the patient can breathe better and sleep more comfortably. For instance, while I was experiencing an attack of sinusitis, I received five treatments in one week (two in one day: night and morning) and my sinuses cleared in six days. I also kept off dairy produce at that time. This was an infection that was dealt with the moment it appeared and was easily despatched. For a long-standing problem it is important to allow a little time between treatments, in order to let the energy stimulated by the candle do its work.

There are always exceptions to every rule, and in my earlier book I mentioned the elderly lady whose niece had used 10 candles in one session and, by the time she had finished, her aunt's hearing had improved dramatically. (See Chapter 2: Age-Related Deafness.)

A therapist in France reported that he used 14 candles on a patient during a demonstration at a health exhibition. This lady wore two hearing aids, and he persuaded her to leave them out for as long as possible. He didn't even need to say that because by the end of the treatment she was hearing without them. When he called her a week later she could talk to him on the telephone, something she hadn't done for years—her hearing aids had been discarded. On checking two years later, he told me that she still hadn't needed to use them again, although I would imagine she has received follow-up treatments during that period. Still, an impressive result. (See Chapter 2: Hearing Aid Wearers.)

I used four candles at one session on a patient, who was also a therapist: she made a specific request, as she had sinus problems.

Three days later she called to say that her nose had just started streaming with a brownish discharge, indicating that there was some very old stuff coming out, although it had taken several days for her body's energy to shift it.

Another example of four candles in one session was for a young man who also had sinus problems. The next day, he reported that he felt wonderful and had been able to sleep on his stomach for the first time in years. Later, due to some difficult circumstances in his life, the blockages crept back. As a therapist himself, he knew who was 'getting up his nose' and what he needed to do to sort things out.

One very interesting example of a multiple treatment happened as I was writing this book, and I just had to include it. A friend of mine woke up one morning with a bad migraine, and she felt generally unwell. Two days later a painful lump formed behind one ear. Her husband did the candles the following evening, which certainly started the ball rolling, although she didn't feel any change at the time. Two days later she came to see me, and I used two candles in each ear to treat her. Twenty-four hours later, when she applied light pressure with a hot towel to the lump, she reported that 'masses of greenish/yellow yucky stuff' oozed out. She said that she then had a wonderful night's sleep and her nasal passages were clearer than they had been for 'longer than I can remember'.

It is important to let the candles do their work. If there has been no immediate change it doesn't mean they haven't been effective, as two of these cases show that it took a few days for the improvement to happen. I would also stress again that any aggravation of the problem afterwards is very normal in complementary therapies. This is due to the fact that healing starts from within and the source of the problem must be corrected first. This runs counter to conventional medicine, which typically suppresses the symptoms and places little emphasis on the underlying cause.

It is also important to emphasize again that an ear candle treatment represents the start of a process rather than an end in itself. As mentioned earlier, when the physical work has stopped, the body's energies continue to benefit from the treatment.

Several years ago, I had an attack of pharyngitis, and despite sulphur inhalations, my sinuses remained blocked. A friend gave me a candle treatment and, as she finished the first side and I turned over, the passages popped open and stayed open. This was another occasion where I received treatment at the start of a temporary condition, so it was easy to treat. As in all complementary therapies, the time needed to heal relates directly to the length of time the person has been suffering: the more long-standing the problem, the more treatments will be needed. I must add, however, that we're all different and I've had some amazing results with just one or two candle treatments.

Conditions that become chronic are a sure sign that the body is seriously out of balance. We may not notice or we may even ignore the small nuisances as they appear. As a rule, people can be divided into those who 'don't make a fuss' and those who rush to consult someone at every opportunity. Neither approach is helpful, and, when we realize that we are developing allergies or suffering from the same problem several times a year, it is advisable to consult a homoeopath or a reputable nutritionist and see what we can do to bring our bodies back into balance.

Combining Candling with Other Therapies

A homoeopathic practitioner who had several patients suffering from tinnitus tried using the ear candles. She explained that homoeopathy had helped with the condition but had been unable to eradicate it completely. The results were much more satisfying when she used the candles in conjunction with a homoeopathic treatment.

An acupuncturist told of a patient who had a swollen lymph gland on her face near one ear. She managed to reduce it with acupuncture, but the patient found that after a night's sleep it was often painful and puffy again. The therapist tried the candles in the hope that they would drain the lymph, and this is exactly what they did. The lump completely disappeared in a very short time.

Reflexology is a treatment that goes well with ear candles. Used first, it can open the body's energy channels, making the effect of the candles more powerful. Working on the meridian (subtle energy) lines of the body, reflexology by itself is a very powerful tool in the therapist's armoury and excellent results have been obtained. For specific conditions where the candles are recommended, the combined treatment acts faster and even more deeply.

Massage practitioners, especially aromatherapists, frequently combine candles with their treatments. Candling is also used in conjunction with colonic irrigation to effect a complete detoxification. There is no end to the combinations that therapists have found to be effective. The candles are used in conjunction with many different methods, enhancing whatever therapy is being practised at the same session.

Contraindications

Perforated eardrum. This has been known to occur in rare cases during syringing. It has also been reported by people who have had their ears 'cleaned' on the beach in India, which is quite common and usually done with a piece of wire. The person doing it will then show you 'what came out of your ear', although I have been told there is some sleight-of-hand involved to make it appear that a large lump of wax has been removed. Apart from the risk of infection, one or two people have reported that it caused the eardrum to bleed. If the eardrum has been perforated it usually heals up quite quickly. If it doesn't, then a cranial osteopath could possibly help. (See Chapters 4 and 6.)

Grommets. This is the same as having a perforated eardrum, but people don't always make the connection. Grommets, which are tube-shaped devices, are used in cases of otitis, or 'glue ear', when the Eustachian tubes (which run from the middle ear) become gummed up by a sticky liquid that becomes infected and the person (usually a child, but more and more an adult), develops a hearing problem. The grommet makes a tiny hole in the eardrum although, once it has fallen out, the drum should close of its own accord. I usually advise waiting 9–12 months from the time the grommets come out before using the ear candles; this gives the eardrum plenty of time to heal. (For more information on this see Chapter 2: Children and Candles, and Chapter 6.)

A recent injury to the head or neck. If there has been a recent injury to the head or neck, it is essential to seek medical assistance and/or to consult an osteopath. I have trained several osteopaths, and they are obviously able to decide at what point the injury has healed and the candles can be used. They have found the therapy to be a very useful addition to their practice.

An allergy to the contents of the candle. This is so rare that I have never come across it. The contents of the candles are used in such minute quantities that I don't see a problem here, but it is as well to keep it in mind.

A child under 12 months of age.

A patient with a cochlea implant.

Eczema in the outer ear. The warmth of the candles would cause it to dry up even more and cause discomfort. **NOTE:** Eczema elsewhere on the body is not a contraindication.

A patient under the influence of recreational drugs or alcohol. Candling could cause a rush of blood to the head and make the patient feel dizzy and nauseous.

According to one source, ear candles could be contraindicated after heavy dental work. If the patient were likely to feel uncomfortable during the treatment, then I agree. However, one of my students told me that she used them on a patient, as she felt they could help in this situation, and when the lady returned to her dentist he was amazed at how quickly the area was healing.

NOTE: Patients are strongly advised not to wash their hair, go swimming, or use iPods, mobile phones, or any source of sound going directly into the ear (land lines being less harmful than mobiles, although not necessarily advisable, either) for the rest of the day following a treatment.

CHAPTER 2

Principal Uses
for the Candles and
Case Histories

Age-Related Deafness

Elderly (or perhaps not-so-elderly) people may find their hearing less acute than it was. Indeed, they are often told by their families and friends that it is so. I can report good results in many of these cases, which have often come about due to a slowing down of the body's energies. A number of treatments may be needed before the patient feels an improvement, but not always: an elderly man told me that after receiving a treatment using just one pair of candles, his hearing had vastly improved. This would, of course, not be the norm, and I do not imagine that this improvement had a lasting effect.

More common is the experience of one therapist I know, who was very keen to try the candles on her elderly father. She started by giving him a treatment once a week; later, she reduced it to once every two weeks, despite his protestations, as he enjoyed the experience very much. After several months, he discovered that not only was he hearing on registers he had been told were lost forever but had no further use for his hearing aid, which now sat unused at the back of a drawer (see also Chapter 1: Multiple Treatments).

As a side note: a study carried out in by Wageningen University and Wageningen Centre for Food Sciences and University Hospital in Maastricht, Holland (Durga, J.,Verhof, P., et al., 2007)[1] found that people between the ages of 50 and 70 receiving folic acid supplements of 800 micrograms per day for three years experienced a lower level of hearing loss than those given a placebo. As well as supplements, folate can also be found in green leafy vegetables, chickpeas, and lentils.

Cancer (see also Chapter 5)

A reflexologist in Switzerland told me how the candles had worked for her mother, who was suffering from terminal cancer. The daughter found an earlier edition of my book, which also contained the chapter on ear candling and cancer therapy. She started treating her with candles and reflexology. After the first treatment, her mother felt less stressed in her stomach and was able to eat and digest more food as the swelling had gone down into her abdomen. Some of her back pain diminished significantly, too, although this could have been due to the stomach being freed from the pressure.

After several weeks of combined treatments, her mother could no longer stand her feet being massaged as, when a person's body is in a terminal state, whether s/he knows it consciously or not, life starts leaving from the feet. However, the candles helped this lady and her daughter continued treatment. In her mother's final days, the candles enabled her to breathe more freely. She felt a huge difference the nights after a treatment, when she was able to sleep reasonably well; the nights she hadn't received a treatment she felt as if she were suffocating. She died a few days before I met the therapist, who told me the candles had been a revelation; she would never have thought they could work at such a deep level.

Candida

C. albicans is a type of fungus that can grow yeast cells and is a causal agent in opportunistic and genital infections in humans. It exists in the bodies of 80 per cent of the human population with no harmful effects, although overgrowth results in candidiasis. This is often observed in immuno-compromised individuals, such as patients suffering from AIDS. It also may occur as a result of chemotherapy, organ or bone marrow transplants, or hospital-acquired infections.

I have been made aware of two cases of candida after candling, and both people were convinced that the candles had caused the infection. The candles cannot, I repeat cannot, cause an infection, but I suspect that what could have happened is this. With the stimulus to the lymph system, the lymphatic fluid had started to drain as it is intended to do. It had got as far as the lymphatic ganglions behind the ears and been blocked from going any farther, possibly by a cervical vertebra being out of alignment. This had then resulted in a candida infection. The first person who consulted me about this confirmed that she had a weak immune system and was using homoeopathy to treat it. The second case was reported to me by someone else, and it was most likely for the same reason. I would suggest trying osteopathy first in such a case.

Goldenseal is a very useful herb for treating candida overgrowth. It promotes the flow of bile and has been found extremely effective against a variety of bacteria, yeast, and fungi, such as *E. Coli*, as well as candida.

Children and Candles

Many children and some adults suffer from *otitis media*, or 'glue ear', as it's more commonly called, at some time in their lives. This is due to a build-up of fluid in the middle ear, which can then become infected. The 'glue' is a sticky fluid that concentrates in the Eustachian tubes, which run from the middle ear (hence the Latin term *otitis media*) down the side of the jaw; the 'glue', can cause pain when the build-up presses against the eardrum. I have been told that the Eustachian tubes in a child run more horizontally than vertically for the first six or seven years of life, this being one of the reasons they are prone to blocking. The 'glue' can be a breeding ground for bacteria, as well as impairing hearing by preventing the vibration of the tiny bones (the ossicles) that conduct sound in the middle ear.

Operations to drain the fluid consist of making a small hole in the eardrum and inserting a tube, or grommet, which keeps the eardrum open and enables the fluid to seep out. Grommets are designed to fall out after several months. (See also Chapter 4.) According to Dr John Briffa, a leading authority on the impact of nutrition and other lifestyle factors on health and illness, writing in his column for the UK *Daily Mail* in 2001, surgery has been found ineffective in improving hearing for longer than six months and may actually worsen it in the long term.

Sometimes one or both grommets fall out almost immediately, the hole closes, and the fluid builds up again; even when the grommets have stayed in place for the required time, the problem can recur a few months later if the underlying cause has not been addressed. I was once consulted by a mother whose child had had five operations and the surgeon was keen to operate again. In around 2–3 per cent of cases, the eardrum has been perforated anyway by the force of the infection.

Dr Gillian Rice, writing on *www.NetDoctor.co.uk*, is of the opinion that around half of all bouts of 'glue ear' will get better spontaneously within three months, and about 95 per cent will do so within one year. As a result, some doctors are reluctant to use any form of treatment unless the 'glue ear' persists for a long period. She also mentions a study showing that half of all children with grommets need to have them reinserted within five years of the initial operation. This gives plenty of time for the parents to find a gentler solution that will solve the problem rather than the symptoms.

This was borne out by a young woman who told me she had had an operation on both ears at a young age and had suffered from migraines and associated problems ever since. If the infection had been given time to clear on its own, she could possibly have avoided the unpleasant consequences of the operation.

According to Patrick Holford and Dr James Braly, authors of *Hidden Food Allergies* (Piatkus, 2006), an important cause of otitis is food allergens. Holford and Braly estimate that at least four out of five children are food allergic, and this causes the Eustachian tubes to swell and close. Once the offending foods have been identified and eliminated from the diet, the tubes will open and drain and any infection will disappear.

There is also a body of evidence showing that routine, repetitive use of antibiotics in treating *otitis media* leads to a three- to six-fold increase in its recurrence. A colleague told me that her three-year-old son had suffered from one ear infection after another and had been given antibiotics each time. She switched to a homoeopathic practitioner, who treated the boy naturally, and from then on, the infections stopped completely. She was also given a list of foodstuffs that he should avoid.

Ear candles have proved to be a great success with young people; they love them, and parents have found that their children ask for the candles when their ears start to feel uncomfortable. When mothers enquire how often they should use them, I suggest they listen to what the child wants, as s/he is the best judge. Of course, if they notice the child is suddenly hearing less well or pulling on the ears, then it's time for a treatment.

A mother and her small son came to a demonstration I gave at a health exhibition in Scotland. He had had many problems with painful ear infections, and his mother wasn't sure he would agree to something else being tried. His behaviour was that of an extremely disturbed child, a result of his pain and suffering. He cowered in a corner as his mother had her ears candled, although she talked to him throughout, explaining that it didn't hurt. She and my colleague were finally able to gain his confidence and get him on the table and his mother gave him the treatment herself, which he even enjoyed. She bought some candles for use at home, and we gave her information on diet.

If a child is scared or reticent about receiving a treatment, seeing a parent or someone they trust being treated first can often do the trick. When it's the child's turn, I demonstrate with the first candle and then supervise the accompanying adult with the second one. This ensures that the person not only feels confident about continuing the treatment at home but also knows how to do it properly.

Although a full candle each side for all ages is the norm, with small children it is possible to extinguish the candle two-thirds of the way down, or to use a cone, as these tend to be shorter; certainly if the child is apprehensive, it is better to do a less lengthy session the first time. The candles need to burn down to the same level each side for the sake of balance, but if children become bored and fidgety by the end of one whole candle, they may say they don't want any more. In the days when I worked at health exhibitions, we marked the candle halfway down and explained to children that we would tell them when we had reached that point, leaving them to choose whether to continue or not: in every case, the child opted for a complete treatment.

More recently, I have treated several small children in my practice and usually burn at least two-thirds of a candle on each side. As mentioned above, cones could be suitable, too, as they are generally shorter. Candle treatments carried out in the calm atmosphere of the treatment room are hugely different from those that take place at a busy health exhibition, where all kinds of energies are swirling around and affect children in particular.

An experience I had with a four-year-old girl in my private practice brought home to me conclusively how effective candling can be on youngsters, especially in the right surroundings. The little girl's mother comes every now and then for a treatment, so she had explained to her daughter what to expect, and the child was quite happy to lie down and hold her mother's hand while I candled her ears. The reason for the visit was that the family was going on a long trip and the girl had a blocked nose and sinuses. By the second candle, she was not only sound asleep but we had to shake her gently to wake her up after around 10 minutes, when she went home in a daze. Her mother later reported that her daughter's nose had been running for two or three days, and after that she was completely clear.

One therapist who bought candles from me during my time in London uses several therapies to treat his many child patients. He told me that he had heard about the candles and initially thought the whole concept rather weird, but then a colleague at the same clinic had explained to him that, yes, they did look odd but they were extremely effective. So he started using them on children suffering from 'glue ear', giving one treatment and showing the mother how it was done so that she could carry on treating at home. When he spoke to me, he was thrilled to recount that two of his child patients had had operation dates to insert grommets cancelled as there was no longer any need for them.

A similar thing happened to one of the therapists I trained in Switzerland. She gave three treatments within the space of a few days to a four-year-old, making sure to get them in before an appointment with a specialist who would be deciding on surgery. When the day arrived and the specialist looked into the little girl's ears, he suggested she come back in six months as nothing needed to be done right away. Her mother had already decided that she would continue with the candles and under no circumstances would her child have an operation.

The role diet plays in illness should never be underestimated, and this is particularly so in the case of children. A link between 'glue ear' and food sensitivity was found back in the 1940s, so it's not new. Now we are seeing more and more allergies to cow's milk and cow's milk products, which are mucus-forming. Other culprits can be wheat, corn, eggs, yeast, and soy.

The finger of blame is usually pointed at the lactose (sugar) in cow's milk, but the problem could be caused by casein, the protein that makes up 80 per cent of that found in cow's milk, which triggers problems with digestion. Milk from goats or sheep is typically more easily digested, even by those who are lactose intolerant; milk from the latter does contain lactose but the proteins are completely different from cow's milk, which may be why it can be tolerated more easily. Unfortunately, it is often the foods we crave or tend to eat regularly that can be problematic.

A team of Finnish researchers reported in the journal *Allergy* (Dunder, T., Kuikka, L., et al., 2001)[2] that children who develop allergies ate less butter and more margarine compared with children who did not develop allergies. They point out that nearly all commercially marketed margarines are made with soy oil. (See also Chapter 3.)

Another factor was brought to my notice by a friend whose granddaughter was milk-allergic and frequently suffered from 'glue ear'. In desperation, her parents took her to an elderly country dweller known for his healing powers. The moment he set eyes on the little girl he pronounced that she had a problem with her ears due, he insisted, to the residues of the vaccines with which she had been injected. I also happen to know that in this case the mother unexpectedly became pregnant very soon after the birth of her first child, and there was some discussion as to whether she would continue with this pregnancy or not. Rather like patients in a coma, unborn babies hear everything. Our hearing is the first sense we develop and the last we lose, and this could certainly have been a factor here.

There is much information on the web involving children and the link between sugar and the immune system, and two studies mentioned on many sites and reported in the *American Journal of Clinical Nutrition* (Sanchez, A., et al., 1973; Bernstein, J., et al, 1997)[3, 4] demonstrate that the ability of white blood cells to kill bacteria is hampered for up to three hours after ingesting 100 grams of sugar (the equivalent of three cans of sweetened soft drink).

Through his prodigious studies on the effects on the ear of xylitol, a sugar substitute that is also mentioned in Chapter 3, Professor Matti Uhari from the University of Oulu in Finland discovered that xylitol chewing gum significantly prevented ear infections in children (Uhari, M., Kontiokari, T., et al., 1996).[5] The Finns have done a great deal of work on natural xylitol and have enabled us to discover more of its benefits for health.

Dr Françoise Berthoud, a Swiss homoeopathic paediatrician, writes in her book *Mon enfant a-t-Il besoin d'un pédiatre?* (Ed. Ambre, 2006) about cases of repeated bouts of 'glue ear', which were successfully treated in the following manner:

1. removing dairy products from the diet;
2. treatment from a chiropractor;
3. draining vaccines with homoeopathy;
4. administration of a homoeopathic remedy; and
5. a child whose deafness stemmed from what she heard while in the womb. Once the mother had understood this and had worked on her own emotions—which caused her to shed floods of tears—at the age of 7, the child was hearing perfectly.

The case of a Down's syndrome child was reported to me, as these children often have very waxy ears. This little girl's mother tried the candles on her; the child loved them, and the next day wax started to seep out. Her mother was delighted to find a gentle remedy that her daughter liked and that would bring some relief, as her excessive ear wax had been an ongoing problem.

Second-hand smoke in the home can be a major culprit in childhood ear infections. Candida may also cause a problem after a course of antibiotics. When a child is screaming with pain, and the ears are waxy, a general practitioner cannot see what exactly is happening and may tend to prescribe antibiotics to be on the safe side, although unfortunately this is likely to compound the problem, as we have already seen.

It has also been found that when mothers are going through a difficult period, their children can develop colds and earaches as a response to this stressful situation—clearly demonstrating the strength of the bond between a mother and her child.

Hazel Courtney, a well-known expert in holistic medicine in the UK, suggests that in cases of 'glue ear', sufferers should eat plenty of carotenoid-rich foods as they keep the immune system healthy. These include spinach, carrots, and sweet potatoes. She also advocates two drops of warm garlic oil in the ear to reduce pain. A little neroli oil dabbed behind the ears has also proved very soothing for children suffering from this problem.

Constipation and Haemorrhoids

Because the candles stimulate the immune system and thus work on the whole body, I have lost count of the number of patients who tell me that the day after a treatment it isn't unusual for them to have several bowel movements. Real constipation can be the result of many factors, however, with long-standing, stubborn constipation requiring several treatments over a short period and possibly combining the candles with other therapies.

It is vitally important for people prone to constipation to drink plenty of water, as dehydration results in hard, dry stools that are difficult to evacuate. They should limit their consumption of caffeinated beverages, such as black tea and coffee; instead, they should drink water, herbal infusions, and freshly squeezed fruit and vegetable juices.

The mother of one of my students, after just one candle treatment, found herself having several bowel movements over the next couple of days—proof, if any were needed, that her immune system had been stimulated and was expelling the waste from her body. Another patient who came for two treatments in a five-day period to get rid of a stubborn infection also reported that the day after the first one she had had three bowel movements. After receiving her first treatment and finding herself having more frequent bowel movements, a lady of 90 was worried until she was told by another patient (a lady of 89) that having several bowel movements after an ear candle treatment is quite normal.

Someone who has come every month for several years, with the exception of July and August, arrived one September morning for a treatment. I had just about finished, when he had to run to the lavatory. Although he had initially come to see if ear candles could help his allergies and keep his sinuses clear rather than his intestines, the effect was immediate.

A patient having problems with haemorrhoids consulted me and I candled her ears. I then burnt a candle over the base of her spine (the sacrum). She stayed fully dressed, and I just placed a paper tissue under the candle to stop any greasy residue staining her clothes. She reported feeling lots of activity in her intestines during the treatment, and the following day she had two bowel movements. Five weeks later she came back for a second appointment and told me she had passed no blood since her first appointment and had had no pain since then, either. (See Chapter 7: Body Candling.)

Something else that she reported to me a month or so after the second treatment was that she was hardly perspiring and had stopped using a deodorant as it felt sticky on her dry skin. That puzzled me at first, but it is easily explained. Toxins are excreted through the skin, and as my patient has a healthy lifestyle, after candling she had far fewer toxins. As a therapist herself, she is used to listening to her body's messages, but some patients might not notice or not make the connection with the treatment.

Ear Infections

Ear candles are recommended for ear infections, as long as the infection is not causing a feeling of dryness and heat: this would be a contraindication. My first line of action would always be a candle treatment, possibly repeated every day for a week or so, to stimulate the immune system sufficiently to clear the condition, as it's only when our immune systems are not functioning as well as they should be that we pick up infections.

It happens to us all at times, to some more than to others. A period of stress, the loss of a loved one, a job, or any situation that throws us out of our comfort zone can have a deleterious effect and pull our defences down, leaving us easy prey for any bug or virus in the vicinity. For someone whose health is normally good, an ear candle treatment every few weeks should be enough to help it stay that way, and I have patients who have been coming regularly for several years who can attest to that.

A link between viruses and the ears was made in the early 20th century. In 1928, Dr Richard Simmons hypothesized that the viruses causing colds and flu enter our bodies through the ear canal and not through the eyes, nose, or mouth as had been commonly supposed. Although he advised keeping fingers out of the ears, most bugs are so microscopic that they can be airborne, and once they enter our inner ears they start to breed and travel anywhere in the body.

Dr Simmons's theories were dismissed; however, Dr Loretta Lanphier, ND, CN, HHP, in an article on www.naturalnews.com supports his theory. She mentions putting a few drops of 3 per cent hydrogen peroxide (H_2O_2) into each ear to treat colds and flu; Greg Webb, RMT, has discovered that remarkable results can be achieved within 12–14 hours by using this method.

Synthetic antibiotics, which are often prescribed for ear infections, should be avoided as much as possible as not only do they work on the symptoms without treating the underlying cause but they also destroy the good bacteria in the gut along with the bad; prolonged courses can adversely affect the digestive system, causing a burning sensation. Several people have mentioned this to me, and I refer to it in the section on clay therapy.

In 2006, *JAMA,* the Journal of the American Medical Association, reported on a trial with 283 children suffering from ear infections who were either given an antibiotic immediately or told to 'wait and see' (Spiro, D.M., et al., 2006).[6] There was no difference between the two groups in terms of pain or fever, yet within the 'wait and see' group those who finally took the drug experienced higher fevers and more ear pain than those who took nothing at all.

A wide variety of natural antibiotics that can clear infections rapidly is available, including (*inter alia*) colloidal silver, garlic, raw propolis, grape seed extract, and Echinacea. Although they only target the 'bad' bacteria and do not destroy the good, one can always combine their use with a course of acidophilus or probiotics to build up the 'friendly' bacteria in the gut. The fact that an infection has taken hold in the first place means that the immune system hasn't been successful in keeping it at bay, so a course of probiotics is recommended. (See also Chapter 4, and the section on Candida in this chapter.) The assistants in a reputable health food shop are well versed in the products they sell and can give you advice about what to buy. You are best advised, as always, to consult a complementary practitioner trained specifically in the use of natural supplements.

Silver is an age-old and very powerful remedy against infection, and with colloidal silver easily available, it now comes in a formula that is easy to administer. It is said that the early settlers who crossed North America would put a silver dollar in their milk churns to stop milk curdling, and it is widely used in centres dealing with victims of burns and in general hospitals to cut the risk of infection.

Colloidal silver has been around for decades and *The Colloidal Silver Report* compiled by Zoe Adams (Another Country Verlag, 2003) is excellent in its citation of studies and its uses. So what is colloidal silver? It consists of nanoparticles of silver suspended in water. After about 12 months the particles fall to the bottom of the bottle and it is no longer effective. I have used it for over 15 years, since I picked up a bug in the office where I worked. The air conditioning had broken down and, when it was repaired, several of us fell ill with sore throats and flu-like symptoms as the bugs and dust in it started to circulate again. At a small health exhibition I found someone selling colloidal silver, and, as I already knew about it and how powerful it was against infections, I took my first dose immediately and by the time I arrived home my sore throat had diminished by 50 per cent. I have continued to use it ever since, and it has never failed me.

A study carried out at the National Taipei University of Technology (Tien, D.C., Tseng, K.H., et al, 2008)[7] on the fabrication of colloidal silver showed that solutions with an ionic silver concentration of 30 ppm or higher are strong enough to destroy *Staphylococcus aureus*, which is an infection that complicates healing in many immuno-deficient patients when it is contracted in hospital. In fact, this infection can be contracted anywhere where people are in confined accommodation, where hygiene may be poor, and/or where people's immune systems are depleted.

Propolis, the antibiotic the bees use to keep their hives sterile, is also extremely effective against infections of all kinds and when taken internally does not interfere with the good bacteria in the gut either. **NOTE:** many people are extremely allergic to bee venom and bee products, so if this is the case, it is important that you try a different remedy.

On the first day of one health exhibition at which I was working, I developed a sore throat and started to lose my voice. At the time I was friendly with another exhibitor who worked with bees and propolis and later became the No. 1 supplier of bee products in the UK. He gave me a bottle of propolis tincture and suggested swallowing it on a tiny piece of bread to coat the throat more thoroughly. The next day I was much better and rapidly back to normal. Be careful, it stains as I can attest, two ruined t-shirts later!

The efficacy of grape seed extract, another powerful natural antibiotic, has been discovered by researchers at the Department of Pharmaceutical Sciences at the University of Colorado Cancer Center in late-stage colorectal cancer (Kaur, M., et al., 2008),[8] according to them, it is more successful than chemotherapy in treating it. Their studies have also shown that it could offer a powerful (and less damaging) alternative to chemotherapy for other types of cancer.

I always keep a bottle of grape seed extract at home. It came in very handy after I had some deep dental work on a gum infection—

waking up in pain in the middle of the night, I took a dose, and the pain disappeared rapidly. I always take grape seed extract on holiday with me, too.

Echinacea is made from the dried juice of the fresh aerial parts and roots of several different species of the plant *echinacea*, also known as coneflower, a beautiful wildflower in the daisy family that is native to North America. It is a very useful herbal product, which traditionally has been used by Indian tribes in North America to reinforce the immune system. For people who feel a cold coming on, or are going to another continent on holiday, it is a good precaution to take Echinacea. Some people consider it a wonder plant for infectious diseases, and it is very effective when working on ear infections such as sinusitis and 'glue ear'. Echinacea is extremely popular in Switzerland, where I live; Dr Alfred Vogel was a Swiss phytotherapist, and his products are very well known, well respected, and available everywhere here. As soon as I or my friends get the sniffles we resort to it and I always take a course before going on holiday to a different environment.

Although honey is not really an antibiotic, I have included information about honey in general in this section, as it is found in many ear candle brands. Active Manuka honey from New Zealand is used by many people for its antibiotic properties. It is extremely powerful and considered to be the purest on the market. It is quite expensive and probably not something you would put on bread as it has a very unusual taste. Honey has been found very effective in the treatment of leg ulcers, and how many of us have drunk hot lemon and honey to soothe our throats when we have a cold and have got rid of the infection at the same time?

In *What's the Alternative* (Boxtree, 1996), UK health expert Hazel Courtney suggests using homoeopathic remedies for ear infections. These include Pulsatilla (30c) or Belladonna (30c), taken every 3-4 hours. If the problem is in the right ear, she recommends *Hepar-Sulph* (30c).

In times gone by, nobody took vitamins, as our food gave us everything we needed. However with the depletion of the soils in which our food is grown and the increase in processed foods, things have changed and we can no longer be sure about the nutritional quality and quantity of our foods. As a result, many people have opted to take supplementary vitamins, in order to absorb the recommended daily amounts (RDAs) of the key vitamins required for health.

One vitamin that is important, for example, is vitamin A, which helps reinforce the immune system. A reply to one reader's query on Lynne McTaggart's *What Doctors Don't Tell You* website, posted by a mother whose child was recovering from an illness, pointed to the fact that the importance of vitamin A has been underplayed, and it has a crucial role in maintaining the smooth functioning of numerous bodily processes. It also helps to regulate the immune system by enabling lymphocytes, the white blood cells that fight infection and disease, to work more effectively.

Although I use natural antibiotics for simple infections and household remedies such as arnica for bruises, I do not take any vitamins or supplements without advice from a practitioner who is well versed in such things. Our bodies are perfectly constructed, and it is important not to dose ourselves with something that sounds as if it could be beneficial without seeing how it is going to affect the rest of the body and whether it could send our system out of balance.

In the 1870s, Dr Wilhelm Heinrich Schüssler found that 12 different types of mineral salt covered all the possible mineral deficiencies in the human body (Jolly, Rajan Singh, 2012).[9] How did he select them? He worked on the basis that these are the salts that remain in the ash when a body has been cremated, and he therefore hypothesized that they must be the basic salts that every cell requires to function normally and to stay healthy. He recommends different salts for different types of ear infection, but the main one for children seems to be *Kalium sulfuricum*. A qualified practitioner would be able to guide you on what to take and when.

In 2000, when I broke my wrist, my physiotherapist recommended that I take *calcium phosphoricum* and silica. She told me that this was not dangerous to take for as long as I wanted. When I found out the effect that the silica at least was having on my hair growth (silica comes from the horsetail plant) I decided to carry on taking it.

These salts are widely prescribed in Switzerland. The best book I've found on the subject is by Gisela Elisabeth Geiger. It is called *Les sels minéraux de Schüssler: Manuel pour se guérir soi-même* (Ed Trédaniel, 2002). **NOTE:** It is available only in German or French.

In *The Complete Book of Water Healing* (Contemporary Books, 2002), Dian Dincin Buchman suggests alternating hot and cold compresses and to relieve any pain, a hot salt bag application. This is made by putting two pounds of coarse sea salt in a cotton pillow case and heating it in the oven. When it's hot, wrap it well in a towel to prevent burning, and lie down with it against the afflicted ear. If there is pus or catarrhal blockage in the ear, the salt will draw the waste out and relieve the pressure. She offers many other ideas for treating ear infections, while insisting on the role food allergies play.

One old-fashioned remedy she mentions in the same book is wrapping a warm clove of garlic in a small piece of cloth (preferably flannel), which has been wetted in hot water and wrung out. The heat and the active ingredients of the garlic will begin to draw out the pain and infection. Repeat as soon as the heat has gone. However, it may be easier and more pleasant to take garlic capsules in fairly high doses. Your local health food shop will be able to advise you on this. When I was working at health exhibitions in the 1990s, on a stand with other practitioners and suppliers, one of the vitamin manufacturers told me that if he developed a cold he took a whole bottle of Kyolic garlic tablets in one day, and that was enough to stop it in its tracks.

Excessive Ear Wax and Poor Hearing

Ear wax (cerumen) is produced as a means of trapping dust, foreign bodies, and so on, preventing them from entering or damaging the ear. It usually makes its own way to the opening of the ear and comes out naturally. As wax is only formed in the outer part of the ear canal, a wax blockage can mean that the individual has been probing his or her ears with foreign objects such as cotton buds and pencils. This only pushes the wax farther in and hardens it, with one of the most common causes for reduction in hearing acuity being a build-up of hardened wax. As mentioned earlier, our ears 'clean' themselves, and we have no need to 'help' the process along.

Although most people have no problem with wax, some individuals do make excessive amounts of it, which can be due to an oversupply of energy in the gall bladder and small intestine meridians. The candles have proved excellent for this condition, as they not only slow down the production of wax but they regulate the rest of the system. From the feedback I have received, they are an important standby for many people.

One early case of excessive wax being successfully treated by ear candles was reported by a colleague. She used candles every two weeks for two or three months, and this regulated the production of wax thereafter. It is worth repeating here that it only takes 24–48 hours to replenish the natural amount of cerumen.

One lady reported that her hearing had been impaired for a while, which she felt was due to an excess of dairy products, including one particular day when she had eaten a huge quantity of ice cream. After using the candles just once, a hard plastic-like lump of wax fell out of one ear and her hearing improved dramatically.

A colleague told me that her husband had had poor hearing for the 10 years she had known him, although he always denied this. When she discovered the candles, she tried them out on the family, and after 9–10 treatments even he had to admit that his hearing was vastly improved as the terrain had been cleaned.

Flying

Many people seek a treatment that can help with the discomfort or even the pain they may experience as an aircraft is depressurizing prior to landing. Some people also have narrower Eustachian tubes, and the pain can build up, especially if the plane is in the air, circling and waiting to land (stacking). The pressure could cause the eardrum to perforate, and although this is rare it has been known to happen. I was a sufferer myself and went through agonies; nothing seemed to help, and I would stuff my fingers in my ears because my ear drum felt as if it would explode at any moment. As I use the candles regularly that is now only an unpleasant memory.

Frequent travellers and business people have found them to be a boon for this reason. The reaction of one of my earliest patients was:

'This is one of the few things I've come across which is supposed to work and which really does'.

A friend whose husband suffered badly and dreaded flying, told me how she had used a pair of candles on him before they took a flight from the UK across the United States to Seattle in the Pacific Northwest. The candles worked wonders, so the couple scoured Seattle, without success, to find another pair to do a further treatment before flying home, although the effects of the first treatment would possibly still have been felt. Had I known more about the candles at that time, I would have suggested that several weeks before flying again she start to give him regular treatments.

Glaucoma

This is a distressing eye condition that is often treated by surgery, but only when it has reached a certain stage. Before that sufferers have all kinds of problems with pressure on the optic nerve and poor vision. According to Dr John Briffa, the most relevant imbalances that may cause it are low thyroid function, food sensitivity, and low adrenal function.

Normally, the tissues at the back of the iris produce an aqueous fluid that occupies the space between the cornea and the lens. Its function is to drain into the bloodstream through the canal of Schlem on the outside of the iris as quickly as it is formed, being replaced every 45 minutes. In the case of glaucoma, the fluid accumulates as a result of poor drainage, and the pressure of its build-up causes pain in the neurons of the retina in the space between the lens and the cornea.

When candles are used, they relax the channels that have become swollen or blocked, thereby enabling the fluid to circulate properly. Having discovered how candling can help glaucoma, I treated a patient with a long-standing condition. After two consultations, she found the pressure in her eyes greatly reduced and, had she lived near me and the treatment continued, we would have achieved an even better and longer-lasting result. (See Chapter 6 for more information.)

Hay Fever, Rhinitis, and Other Allergies

Many of us love the warm days and short nights in summer when we can eat in the garden or picnic in the park, but for some people it is not a happy time at all. People who dread the spring with the trees coming into bloom, or summer with its scent of newly cut grass. Or those who may have an allergy to a foodstuff that they love but dare not eat. These are the sufferers from hay fever and various seasonal allergies, which cause streaming eyes and a blocked nose—often headaches, too. Even in town they are still exposed to the pollen from trees, as well as pollution. Someone whom I know slightly and who is affected by chestnut blossom can, in particularly bad years, suffer for many weeks until the season is finally over.

Another factor leading to allergic rhinitis or asthma is the hypochlorite-based water purifier used in commercial swimming pools to combat body bacteria due to people not showering thoroughly before entering. This type of water purification combines with the creatinine and urea in sweat and urine to form allergens that can cause allergies as well as skin complaints, conjunctivitis, and so on.

A less well-known cause is a group of conditions called non-allergic rhinitis, caused by hormones and occupational factors. This should be checked out seriously. Kinesiology (a form of diagnosis using muscle testing) can be very helpful in pinpointing allergies. Food additives can be responsible, as can chemical cleaning products used in the home. There are less toxic alternatives to the latter and it's worth checking them out. (See Chapter 3.)

A young man in London who was studying to be a doctor and who helped his father in a local shop told me he suffered badly from hay fever. He was interested in alternative therapies; in fact, he was the only student in his year taking an extra course to learn more about them. He bought a pair of ear candles to try and was really impressed with the results, after just one treatment. He assured me it was something he was going to investigate further. (See also Chapter 3.)

In the first human study of its kind, carried out in 2008, scientists at the Institute of Food Research found that *probiotic* bacteria in a daily drink could modify the immune system's response to grass pollen, a common cause of seasonal hay fever (Ivory, et al., 2008).[10]

One of the researchers explained that the *probiotic* strain they tested changed the way the body's immune cells respond to grass pollen, restoring a more balanced immune response.

Ear candles alone are not necessarily going to take away the sensitivity to all these things, but they can make life much more bearable by helping to relieve some of the stuffiness and, used in conjunction with probiotics, can possibly go far in clearing the allergy.

Allergies may have psychosomatic links. One of my professional candling students explained how her son had developed and been cured of an allergy to a particular type of tree. The start of the problem dated back to a day when they were outside surrounded by these trees and something she said gave him a shock. Immediately afterwards, he developed an allergy but nobody made the connection. Many years later, when they traced its source to that day and the particular shock the young man had received, they discussed the matter in question. After that, the allergy disappeared as quickly as it had come.

Hearing Aid Wearers

People using hearing aids can benefit from ear candling (see Age-Related Deafness at the beginning of this chapter), but it's important to discontinue use of hearing aids for as long as possible after candling because the burning of the candles, as mentioned previously, is in itself the start and not the end of the treatment. As an example, during one of the first demonstrations I did at a health exhibition, I candled a lady wearing two hearing aids. As I saw her inserting them again afterwards, I realized the treatment was unlikely to be successful, as putting the hearing aids back into her ears immediately was going to block the energy we had got circulating with the ear candles. The example in Chapter 1: Multiple Treatments seems much more logical.

I had a patient in early middle age for a couple of years. She started with three treatments fairly close together and then came every six to eight weeks. She no longer needs the hearing aid she used to wear in one ear and has turned the sound down on her television. She is absolutely delighted and seems more self-assured.

She told me that if she doesn't hear what someone says (and it happens to all of us sometimes, except that people without hearing problems don't take particular notice of it), she just asks the person to repeat it. I've discovered that the hearing-aid business is extremely lucrative, but however sophisticated (and expensive) the apparatus is, obviously nothing can replicate the body's natural hearing mechanism.

Nowadays, it seems extraordinary to me that we don't realize how unnatural it is to put an object into the body to improve its functioning. The body's wisdom is absolute, and whenever something stops working properly, we should automatically want to know why rather than resorting to drugs, surgery and appliances to solve the problem. Until I worked with body therapies, and especially the ears, when I came into contact with hearing aid wearers, this fact would never have crossed my mind.

People who use ear pieces for any reason (iPods, mobile phones, and so forth) should keep them scrupulously clean and never share them with anyone else, as passing them from one person to another can result in infection to the outer ear. A study of bacterial growth with earphone use was carried out at the Kasturba Medical College in India (Mukhopadhyay, C., Basak, C., et al., 2008).[11] In the group of heaviest users, bacteria were found in ear swabs taken from 23 users (92 per cent) and in earphone swabs from 17 users (68 per cent). This advice also applies to ear plugs, which should only be used on very rare occasions—they can become habit forming, as mentioned earlier. Ear plugs and ear pieces should always be properly disinfected after each use.

Listening to MP3 players at high volume also increases the risk of deafness in later life, warns Professor Peter Rabinowitz of the Occupational and Environmental Medicine programme at Yale University, who has intensively studied noise and its effects. In an article published in the *British Medical Journal* (Rabinowitz, 2010),[12] Rabinowitz states that more than 90 per cent of young people listen to portable music devices such as iPods. He added that inserting earphones into the ear canal intensifies the volume, which can reach over 120 decibels, equivalent to the noise from a jet engine.

Mastoid Discomfort

People who have had an operation on the mastoid portion of the temporal bone just behind the ear can also suffer badly with a build-up of wax. This condition often results from an untreated infection, and the bone needs to be scraped under anaesthetic. Sufferers often complain of frequent headaches that occur throughout their lives.

I shall never forget one of the first patients I treated at my first health exhibition, when I knew very little about ear candles. The results I obtained using candles on this particular lady were amazing. She was a fellow exhibitor at the show and came to see if candling might help her. Plagued by ear problems since childhood, after having an operation for mastoiditis, she suffered constantly and, although she had received all sorts of treatment, nothing had helped her.

With much trepidation on both sides, we went ahead with the candles. A couple of hours later, she came back to my stand to say that wax was 'pouring' out of her bad ear and, as she had short hair and was working with the public, it was most embarrassing. Was there something that would stop it? We explained to her that this needed to happen, and when I saw her six months later she told me how, having used the candles again in the meantime, she had cleared the problems that had affected her all her life, pronouncing the treatment 'heaven-sent'.

Still on the same subject, another customer at a much more recent health exhibition told me she had used the candles several times on her partner. Not only had they helped clear the build-up of wax and debris that had plagued him since his operation for mastoiditis but his epilepsy was vastly improved, too. **NOTE:** I hesitate to make any pronouncements about the effectiveness of candling for those who suffer from epilepsy, as I have little information on the subject. I mention it here in passing only. Great care should obviously be taken with someone who suffers from this condition, and treatment should never, ever be given during a crisis.

Migraines and Headaches

Migraines and headaches have to rank with toothache as the pain that is the hardest to bear. Backache sufferers would probably disagree, but there is a jangling agony, often nausea and vomiting, and a whole range of horrors attached to pains in the head that make them so unbearable.

People who experience regular migraines are invariably on the lookout for something—anything—that can help them. A combination of treatments is probably the best option, but the candles have proved to be very useful indeed in alleviating migraines.

Migraine sufferers usually have certain triggers that tell them an attack is on the way. This is the moment (if possible) to do a candle treatment and encourage the person to sleep afterwards. One patient reported that whenever she was able to do this, several hours later, when she awoke, her migraine had passed.

The wife of a regular migraine sufferer reported that her husband, who had an extremely healthy lifestyle, had come across an old book (now out of print and off the radar) entitled *You Can Heal Your Migraine*. The author advised eating something every three hours, never going hungry, and never having sugar in any form; only honey and maple syrup were permitted. Following this advice, her husband's migraines stopped completely.

It is worth remembering that migraines are connected to the function of the gall bladder, which is why people often vomit; they are not 'digesting' something, possibly mentally as well as physically, and it all has to come out.

Peppermint oil is very soothing, because peppermint helps the digestive system: a cup of peppermint or chamomile tea can either settle the stomach or induce vomiting, thereby releasing some of the pressure.

An old favourite is the herb feverfew. According to a study carried out 25 years ago by Dr E. Stewart Johnson, then director of the City of London Migraine Clinic (Johnson, E.S., Kadam, N.P., Hylands, D.M., et al., 1985), [13] eating 1–5 leaves of feverfew a day, chopped and put into a sandwich, worked as a preventive measure for seven out of 10 patients, causing them to have fewer attacks of lower intensity; one-third of patients had no further attacks at all. One or two of the patients reported having a sore mouth from eating the leaves, but feverfew is available in tablet form, which is a lot simpler, especially for those allergic to gluten who do not eat wheat-based bread. A more recent study was carried out in Germany (Diener, H.C., Pfaffenrath, V., et al., 2006).[14] The team obtained a positive result for those who had received the feverfew against those given a placebo.

Some migraines are brought on by stress or suppressed anger. If this is the case, it is important to note what sets off migraines and why. There are many courses in breathing and relaxation, and books and specially recorded CDs can be helpful for people who feel the need to stay with a situation that causes them stress or frustrates them.

Maintaining regular sleep patterns is important, as is exercise and, of course, attention to diet. Although there are several classic 'no-nos', such as chocolate, cheese, and so on, most migraine sufferers are aware of which foods cause them problems. As mentioned above, it is important not to go hungry, and breakfast in particular should never be skipped. Dehydration plays a role in bringing on a migraine headache, so although it is important for everyone to drink no fewer than 2 litres of filtered water every day, it is even more necessary if you are plagued with migraines.

A vast body of research has been carried out on migraine sufferers and magnesium deficiency. Magnesium relaxes muscles and, as it does so, it may reduce spasms in the blood vessel walls, which are thought to play a part in migraine. **NOTE:** The Feingold Diet has been shown to be very helpful. For more information, visit *www. feingold.org*.

Migraine sufferers are twice as likely to have heart attacks as non-sufferers, according to a study published in 2010 by researchers at Albert Einstein College of Medicine of Yeshiva University in Neurology (Bigal, M.R., Kurth, T., Santello, N., et al., 2010).[15] They also found that migraine sufferers had an increased possibility of suffering a stroke and were more likely to have key risk factors for cardiovascular disease, including diabetes and high blood pressure.

Geneva therapist Michel Bontemps is a fervent believer in what is known as sympaticotherapy. This ancient therapy works on the sympathetic nervous system. It is a form of nasal reflexology, using a small probe topped with a silver ball (sometimes wrapped round with cotton and dipped in essential oils) on the reflex points situated inside the nose. Although this practitioner uses a variety of therapies, he has found that after only three sessions of nasal therapy, combined with cranial osteopathy, patients have reported excellent results. In his experience, nine out of 10 migraine patients have restrictions in the cervical vertebrae, and he is convinced that this treatment will effect a long-term if not definitive cure.

Anyone suffering from a blocked nose and frequent headaches can try dipping a cotton bud into a weak mixture of essential oils and placing it in the nostrils to be inhaled. This can provide great relief.

Another ear candle user told me she had been in a car accident several years previously and every now and then experienced a terrible pain at the back of her head. She had tried everything, but found that only the candles could give her relief. She spoke to me in the very early days, but now I would certainly check that she had tried cranial osteopathy, which is particularly good in the aftermath of trauma from accidents.

My personal experience in treating migraines with candles was with a colleague who suffered from migraines several times a month. She came for three treatments over a period of six weeks and felt a migraine come on during the third one. She came back for a treatment a year later, and as I looked over her notes I asked her about her migraines. She astounded me by saying that not only had she had one solitary attack six months earlier, when she was under a great deal of stress, but she had forgotten why she'd consulted me in the first place!

One therapist suggests a psychosomatic link for migraines, noting that in her experience they often occur in people who did not have a well-balanced start in life: for example, if one parent wanted a child but the other didn't, or if one parent had been emotionally or physically distant. She explained that 'mi-grain' means just that, half the seed. There was an echo of this in the case I have just reported and it very possibly had something to do with the migraines this lady suffered.

Painful Periods

One of my students candled a young girl who suffered from extremely painful periods. She started with a gentle head massage to relax her and, while the first candle burnt, the girl fell into a deep sleep. Her mother persuaded the therapist to let her rest and not to wake her up to work on the other ear as the pain had disrupted her sleep pattern. That evening, the therapist spoke to the girl, who agreed to have a complete treatment the next day. At the end of the second treatment her pain had completely disappeared and she asked the therapist to continue the following month.

My own experience of working on painful periods took place at an open day at a local health clinic, where people could drop in and try out various therapies free of obligation and free of charge. A teenage girl came to try the ear candles and just so happened to be suffering from period pains. As I candled both her ears and gave her some Reiki, the cramps greatly diminished, and she was impressed. I would have liked to treat her again and, had I been able to follow up with her as a regular patient, I may have suggested burning a candle in her navel. (See Chapter 7: Body Candling, for a description of this procedure and a note of caution on performing it.)

Although many factors, from stress (in family or school situations) to poor nutrition, can be involved when it comes to period pains, it's important to note that young women are also dealing with the passage from childhood to womanhood. This can be very traumatic, especially nowadays when little girls are sexualized earlier and earlier, and also in certain societies when the start of menstruation is often a signal that the girl is ready to marry. A homoeopathic practitioner can be very helpful here, as every patient is seen as an individual and treatments are tailored to the person, not the symptoms. If the candles offer relief from the pain, as seems to be the case, then they can be considered an excellent support.

Relaxation

When I was first told that German psychotherapists sometimes use ear candles on their patients before a session to calm them down, I treated the information merely as hearsay and didn't use it. Then, years later, someone who had worked at a centre for adults with learning difficulties in the UK reported that an aromatherapist visited once a week and often used ear candles. The treatment was very popular and highly successful, as it produced a calming effect on the patients.

When I was looking for a professional illustration of a person receiving a candling treatment to use on my literature, I was referred to a graphic artist who had never seen ear candles before and thought them rather a joke. I left him a pair of candles, and he promised to come up with something. When I saw him a couple of weeks later, he was puzzled: 'Are those things supposed to make you sleep?' he asked. I replied that they suited most people as a bedtime treatment. Apparently his partner had done the treatment late one evening, and he had slept very deeply that night. He just wondered if there was a connection…

A therapist, who came on a course, gave and received a treatment and told me that a couple of hours later she was dozing off every now and then and had a wonderful night's sleep. The following day (a Sunday), she was still dozing and began to feel slight pain in her joints, as well as from where she had broken a collar bone years before and an ankle she had sprained. On Monday, she felt better and was astonished that the treatment had stirred up these old wounds. She realized she should be taking better care of herself.

A patient suffering from constant back pain as a result of an accident many years earlier received a candle treatment at a health exhibition on a day when his back was particularly painful. He reported afterwards that during the treatment he could feel the muscles in his lower back relaxing, attenuating his pain, with the effect maintained the following day.

A single treatment at difficult moments is all that is necessary to relieve stress, although this will not be lasting if the causes for the stress are not addressed. I have patients who consult me every now and then for this very reason. I explain that if one treatment triggers any health problems, then they should let me know, so that together we can investigate what is going on. Some patients come from countries where candling is a mainstream therapy and that makes them more open to receiving a treatment now and then as they are more aware of its benefits than many Europeans. For some patients it's rather like having an occasional massage.

Sinus Problems

Sinusitis, or infected sinuses, can be a painful and unpleasant complaint; some people find that every time they develop a cold it affects their sinuses. Dairy products made from cow's milk are heavily implicated in sinusitis, as cow's milk products create extra mucus in the body—the last thing a sinus sufferer needs. Milk, cheese, and yoghurt made from cow's milk are particularly mucus-forming. Sometimes, allergies to other foods, such as wheat and soy, are to blame, so it is worthwhile checking for these, too.

It is important to ensure that teeth are in good condition, as this can affect the sinuses. A friend who had a piece of tooth that broke off and entered the maxillary sinus had to have it removed under general anaesthetic. (See also Tinnitus.)

Steam inhalation of essential oils will help with the congestion, as the correct oils will produce a very soothing effect. Try inhaling the steam from a bowl of very hot water to which has been added three drops of rosemary and one each of thyme and peppermint. Use a towel over the head to keep the heat in. When I was a child we knew nothing of essential oils and always used a preparation called Friar's Balsam. Its base is tincture of benzoin, and it doesn't smell very pleasant, but it was comforting and, more importantly, it worked.

Bowel toxicity is something that has come to the fore in the last 20 years. This is really auto-intoxication by the faecal matter in the large intestine. One of its main effects is sinus congestion, so a sufferer from chronic sinus problems should look at the possibility that his/her bowels are causing or exacerbating the condition. This can be managed very successfully by certain herbal mixtures, fasts, colonic irrigation or liver flushes. It goes without saying that all of these techniques need to be overseen and/or carried out by a qualified practitioner.

During a demonstration of candling at one health exhibition, a lady who was plagued with sinus problems decided to try a candle treatment. She came back to the stand a couple of hours later not looking happy at all. 'You've set off a sinus attack,' she said accusingly, adding that she had a streaming nose and a headache. I wanted to tell her that this was an excellent result, which it indeed was, but it didn't seem to be the right moment! As she had bought a packet of 10 candles, I recommended that she have another treatment that night or the next day and told her that this would help resolve many of the issues she was experiencing.

So what was happening here? As mentioned earlier, with all alternative therapies, it is possible to feel worse at first (this is known as a 'healing crisis') although, once that passes, the problem rarely recurs and if it does, it has much less force. This is extremely common, especially with a long-standing problem, but although I *always* point out this eventuality to patients, they don't necessarily take in the information; as a result, some people are convinced that the ear candle treatment has made their condition worse. For people who are used to starting to feel better as soon as they have popped a pill, this can be distressing, and they are apt to see it as a sign that it is this unconventional treatment that has caused them harm. Nothing could be farther from the truth: it is proof that the body has retained the capacity to excrete some of the toxins that lie at the root of their ill health and it is beginning the self-healing process.

During a more recent health exhibition, I agreed to treat a fellow exhibitor who had had no sense of smell or taste for three months. I gave him several candle treatments over a period of 10 days and his senses started to awaken. Had he been treated earlier, it would certainly have happened faster.

Operations to drain the sinuses are sometimes performed for bad cases of sinusitis. I have met one or two people who have had this surgery but have been dissatisfied with the results; indeed, one friend was even told by her surgeon that the procedure would need to be repeated 10 years later! Meanwhile, she received no dietary guidance as a follow-up to surgery. Eliminating dairy produce (and giving up smoking) would likely have been very helpful in improving her condition. It really is a pity when the first recourse in allopathic medicine is to take the route of medication or surgery, as so many problems of every sort can be alleviated by one or more of the hundreds of gentler complementary therapies now available.

For sinusitis sufferers, the psychosomatic connection (something or someone 'getting up your nose'), should not be neglected, either. For example, a friend found she no longer suffered from sinusitis after she moved out of the family home, where she and her mother were frequently at loggerheads. Too much pressure or feeling stifled by life, any challenging situation or problem involving a loved one can also 'get up your nose'.

Skin Disorders

Ear candles can have a beneficial effect on skin problems, such as an excessively greasy skin, juvenile acne, and circulatory disorders that result in red patches. Following her first treatment, one patient told me how delighted she was with the effect candling had had on her face and scalp, saying that her skin was less greasy and her scalp didn't itch nearly as much. A recent tattoo also healed much faster than the others she had had before. She received two further treatments, and now she frequently contacts me to purchase candles to use on her friends and at home.

Sleep Apnoea

Sleep apnoea involves an interruption in sleep, when the patient suddenly stops breathing for a short period of time and is woken up by his/her autonomic system in distress. Put more simply, the patient snores loudly and suddenly there is a pause when breathing stops. It is very distressing, not only for the sufferer but for anyone who sleeps in the same room; the snoring keeps them awake, and when breathing stops they wait for it to start again (or not). I candled one lady for sleep apnoea who had been issued with an oxygen mask to place over her face before going to bed, the standard medical treatment for the condition. This effectively stopped her from sleeping, anyway. On the day of her consultations she was invariably exhausted on returning home and dozed for several hours. After her third appointment, she went on holiday with her daughters, during which time they shared a bedroom. The girls remarked that their mother's snoring had greatly diminished and the pauses between breaths were shorter. She also confirmed that her constant diarrhoea had abated and she had returned her oxygen machine to her doctor. Her comment after the fourth treatment was: 'Who would think that a simple little candle could have such an effect?'

Inspired by this positive result, one of my ototherapy students decided to treat a man suffering from sleep apnoea as one of her case studies. He had various other health problems, and he also used an oxygen mask for sleeping. The night after the first treatment, he felt very thirsty and drank a lot of water but didn't need the oxygen mask to assist with his breathing. As a heavy smoker and coffee drinker, his body was completely dehydrated, and the effect of the candles enhanced his desire for water. By the third treatment, he was sleeping much less during the treatment and much more at night, and several of his other symptoms—reduced hearing levels, tinnitus, and rhinitis—had improved as well. He felt much calmer and more peaceful, which was probably also due to his sleep patterns reverting to normal.

I would add a note of caution here. I would not recommend that someone who suffers from sleep apnoea and has been prescribed an oxygen mask for night-time use give up using it immediately after their first candle treatment. If the person sleeps alone, s/he may not be able to gauge when it is possible to discard the mask. Many more treatments might be needed to improve this serious health condition. The two success stories above are just examples of what is possible.

Stress Relief

A therapist working on a nearby stand at my very first health exhibition decided to try the ear candles. I heard later from a mutual friend that this girl had been going through a relationship break-up and the day after the treatment she spent a good few hours crying tears not of pain but of release, feeling very much helped in the process. Another, much more recent patient, who had a whole catalogue of effects after the first treatment, also reported a bout of crying with a feeling of relief afterwards. She now comes regularly and tells me that the day after a treatment she feels as if she's been on holiday!

One of my students, who at the time of her training was dealing with a few family problems, found that after her initial ear candle treatment she spent three days crying without knowing why and feeling very tired and depressed. After that she felt greatly at peace.

A therapist I trained told me that she had treated a patient with an extremely stressful life who suffered from tinnitus. It was too early to tell if the ear candles could help his condition as he had had it for a long time, but a few hours after the treatment he was crying floods of tears—a first step in his healing process.

These cases are classic examples of a healing crisis. Each person was suffering from stress or an emotional problem (possibly without even being aware of it), and each person felt the release that the tears brought. However, without knowing that this can happen, patients may be surprised and upset that it has occurred after candling, thinking the candles 'caused' it, or maybe not even making the connection. It also illustrates that the body's energy knows what needs treating first, and the relief of stress in these patients demonstrated that it was the first priority.

From case studies my students present, I have particularly noticed that not only have many of their patients reported feeling calmer but on a few occasions they have found the courage to say something that probably needed saying but which they had been too embarrassed to say earlier.

One patient came to see me suffering with tinnitus brought on by stress. It had started 10 years earlier, when she was taking exams, and had only stopped during her maternity leave from her high-powered job. I explained that the candles could offer relaxation, but the underlying problem would need a different approach, then gave her a foot and leg massage, and candled her ears. Three days later, she reported that not only had she had a wonderful night's sleep but her head felt pounds lighter. I would expect, though, that once she was back in the rhythm of work, this effect would have worn off.

Swimming and Diving

People who love swimming, especially divers, often find their favourite hobby upsets the balance of the inner ear and are extremely prone to ear infections and related problems. Many people I've treated who have had these problems report being helped by the candles, but one person I particularly remember.

While I was demonstrating candling at the Healing Arts Exhibition in London in 1991, a lady stood watching in amazement, saying she had never seen the candles used in public before. It transpired that she had a beauty clinic in the West Indies. People, who had come on vacation to revel in the warm waters of the Caribbean, had consulted her about water lodged in their ears and pressure problems after a lot of swimming and diving, which was spoiling their expensive holidays. An elderly islander showed her how to make ear candles, telling her that people there had always used them. She tried them, obtained excellent results, and continued to use them.

A rather sceptical friend came to me for a candle treatment once after water had become lodged in one of her ears while she was washing her hair. She was unimpressed with the fact that she didn't feel better during the treatment, or immediately afterwards, but contacted me a few days later to tell me that when she had taken a short flight, as the plane gained height, her ear had 'popped' and opened. When the first treatment makes no apparent difference, persuading a sceptical patient that more appointments are indicated can present a challenge.

Tinnitus (Ringing or Other Noises in the Ear)
(see also Chapters 3 and 4)

There can be so many causes for tinnitus, an annoying condition of constant ringing and noise in the ears that can, at its worst, drive people into depression, and even to develop suicidal tendencies. Because there *are* so many causes of tinnitus, there are indeed many factors to look at and I will not pretend that ear candles can cure tinnitus on their own. What I can say is that I have had some positive results using candles, especially when they are combined with other treatments.

I was consulted by someone who had had an accident in childhood and then spent several years working at fairgrounds where noise levels tend to be high. He had undergone an operation on one ear and had suffered from tinnitus ever since. At first I had a long talk with him on the telephone and convinced him to try other therapies: where there's physical damage the candles can offer little help. To my amazement, a few months later he contacted me again and came in for a few treatments. As I thought, there was very little progress, although, with the stimulation of his energy flow, his hearing improved. The only possible suggestion I could offer was the TinniTool® which is a soft laser developed in Switzerland and reputed to be successful in treating tinnitus. I gave him the literature to read, and I really hope that, if he tried it, he was helped because his life was being made miserable by the noise. The last time I saw him he burst out with: 'I wish I'd *never* had that operation'. We can all be wise after we've made a choice that later proves not to have been a good idea, but I think his problem went further back than that.

It's important to note that because the middle ear contains several small bones (ossicles) that can easily be displaced by a long-forgotten, even trivial incident, tinnitus sufferers would be well advised to consult a cranial osteopath before trying other therapies. (For more information, see Chapter 4: Cranial Osteopathy/Craniosacral Therapy.)

I have received innumerable reports of people who were greatly helped by the candles, and others responding better to a combination of candles and other therapies. One patient whom I would dearly have loved to see again came to me suffering from tinnitus. We did the first treatment, then the following week she came back and said her tinnitus had completely disappeared! However, I warned her to be prudent and, in fact, after the second treatment it had come back slightly in one ear. I had explained at the start that three treatments would show whether the candles could help her or not (I did *not* say that only three treatments would be necessary), so we did a third treatment. After that, I didn't see her again. That is a classic example of someone likely to contend that the candles don't work, whereas if she had persevered—and she had been suffering for quite a while—I'm convinced we would have obtained an excellent result.

A student who several months earlier had been the subject of a case study by a fellow student told me that with regular use of the candles her tinnitus had disappeared; it now only comes back slightly when she is extremely tired. As she was a therapist herself, she was more able to see the necessity for perseverance than the above-mentioned patient.

In his book *Tinnitus* (Thorsons, 1986), now sadly out of print, Arthur White, N.D., D.O., makes a strong link between catarrhal disorders and tinnitus. He is a firm proponent of letting colds, catarrh, and fevers run their course, with no input from drugs. In his opinion, if the toxic build-up is not allowed to come out it often leads to tinnitus, as the poisons are forced back into the body before breaking out again in a stronger form. Incidentally, I have noted that the ear candles are at their most effective when excessive catarrh is a problem for tinnitus sufferers.

A more recent piece of information I have found on one of the causes of tinnitus comes from research on the connection between mobile phones and tinnitus, reported in *Occupational and Environmental Medicine* (Hutter, H.P., Moshammer, H., Wallner, P., et al., 2010).[16] The researchers discovered that using a mobile phone for only 10 minutes increased the risk of developing tinnitus by 71 per cent. Many sufferers reported their problem as being on the left side, where they held their phone, and 29 per cent also reported suffering from vertigo.

In 1989, I met an acupuncturist in France who told me he was seeing many cases of kidney problems that resulted from loud personal stereos, as the ears and kidneys are in the same meridian line of the body according to the traditional Chinese system of medicine; they refer to the ears as the flowers of the kidneys. This leads us to the obvious conclusion that if the kidney energy is depleted (and excessive protein, salt or aspirin can have this effect), that will automatically affect the ears, too. According to traditional Chinese medicine, cold has a damaging effect on the kidneys. From my perspective, it's logical to conclude that the warm energy from the ear candle will help to revitalize the kidneys and help to solve hearing problems.

In his best-selling book *Spontaneous Healing* (Ballantine, 2000), well-known US holistic physician Andrew Weil mentions a German doctor working in a hospital devoted to psychosomatic medicine who has had great success treating tinnitus. In the German doctor's opinion, this often comes from chronic muscle tension in the head and neck, usually associated with poor body posture and stress. He has found that yoga and training in relaxation, together with bodywork, frequently enables patients to get rid of this condition permanently.

On the more extreme end of therapeutic options for tinnitus, in his book *Healing in the 21*ˢᵗ *Century,* (Mainstream Publishing, 2001), author Jan de Vries writes at length about the practice of bloodletting using leeches, which was much used in bygone times for all types of illness. Leeches make a small hole and suck out the diseased blood. In their salivary glands, they have very specific enzymes that dilute and detoxify the blood. Many years ago, a colleague told me about a pharmacist who would sell her customers a leech for this reason. Why am I telling you this? According to de Vries, one of the many indications for using leeches is for people suffering from tinnitus, and there are now courses on how to apply them. To treat tinnitus, a leech would be placed behind the ear.

Bloodletting is still practised by acupuncturists in the form of cupping, which involves making small cuts on the skin and placing a warmed glass over them to form a vacuum and draw out the 'bad' blood. This blood is darker and thicker than normal and, in Asian traditions, is thought to cause blocks that can lead to many of the illnesses from which we suffer today. As for leeches, a nurse told me very recently that they are still widely used in hospitals to treat haematomas, carefully covered so that patients can't see these segmented worm-like blood suckers on their skin!

Antibiotics, anti-inflammatories, aspirin, and other medication can lead to whistling in the ears. Tinnitus can also be linked to zinc deficiency. (See Chapter 3: Ototoxic Medication.) Something else that is said to help a tinnitus sufferer is taking high daily doses of vitamin B12. Award-winning health journalist Susan Clark writes in her excellent 'dictionary' *What Really Works in Natural Health* (Bantam Press, 2004) that she is a firm proponent of this but insists on natural products made by a reputable company and advises avoiding synthetics at all costs. I would add that if you want to try this, it is important to check first on whether taking mega doses of vitamin B12 is suitable for you.

Noni juice, which comes from the *Morinda citrifolia* plant, has been found to be very effective for tinnitus. A sufferer writing in Lynne McTaggart's newsletter *What Doctors Don't Tell You* (WD-DTY) reported that after trying almost every natural remedy without success, she discovered that drinking noni juice for four weeks produced an improvement of around 75 per cent. However, do beware of noni juice that isn't 100 per cent pure; only buy organic.

According to Dr H. J. Roberts, in his book *Aspartame Disease: An Ignored Epidemic* (Sunshine Sentinel Pr. Inc, 2001), the artificial sweetener aspartame (E.951), which was discovered by a researcher in a lab whilst seeking a remedy for ulcers and is today included in most ready meals and diet drinks, has proved to be a major factor in cases of tinnitus and has been mentioned in connection with many other health problems. Aspartame contains phenylalanine, aspartic acid, the methyl ester that immediately becomes free methyl alcohol or methanol. According to Dr Roberts, after prolonged storage or being subjected to heat, the components break down and are potentially toxic to the brain and the inner ear. There is a massive body of evidence attesting to its toxicity—so much, in fact, it is difficult to know where to start!

Aspartame goes under several different names (Canderel, Nutrasweet, Equal, and so on), and it is also found in literally hundreds of supermarket products, so checking labels is essential. When a product is labelled as containing 'zero sugar', it is obvious that an artificial sweetener has been used and it's invariably aspartame. This is something that should have been taken off the market long ago, but unfortunately it has some powerful friends. (See also Chapter 3.) Dr Roberts' work has been featured on the website of Dr Betty Martini, D.Hum, who founded Mission Possible World Health International (*www.mpwhi.com*).

A student told me recently that she had a tooth that was bothering her, and finally it got so bad that she went to the dentist. There was an infection under a very old amalgam filling, and as the whole tooth was in bad shape he extracted it. What startled her was that the tinnitus she had had in that ear stopped, as if someone had thrown a switch. Dr John Roberts, a holistic dentist working in the UK, has found that removing amalgam fillings cures many niggling health problems in his patients, including tinnitus. His work is quoted by Deanne Pearson, a holistic health adviser writing in *Here's Health* magazine in November 2001. Dr Roberts reported that one root canal filling produced a charge of half a volt, enough to power a small light bulb! (The importance of healthy teeth is also mentioned in the section on sinus problems.)

From a *What Doctors Don't Tell You* (*www.wddty.com*) newsletter, I discovered that another reader was suggesting the temporomandibular joint (TMJ) could be causing the problem and advised consulting a dentist specializing in bite correction to address this condition.

In 2002, Morgenstern and Bierman published the results of a trial of the herb gingko biloba special extract EGb 761 on 60 patients with chronic tinnitus (Morgenstern, C., Biermann, E., 2002).[17] The test subjects on EGb 761 showed significant improvement compared with those receiving the placebo. A secondary outcome was that there was a decrease in hearing loss and improved self-assessment of subjective impairment. Please do bear in mind that if you are taking blood-thinning drugs, gingko biloba may not be suitable and a physician should be consulted first. A well-researched article published on the web by the University of Maryland Medical Center gives more information on gingko biloba and the uses to which it can be put.[18]

Another useful book that contains a section on tinnitus as well as a case history is an encyclopaedia of alternative healing methods. *How to Stay out of the Doctor's Office* (Instant Improvement Inc. 1992) gives a definition of nearly 60 ailments with a list of probable causes and conventional treatments. There then follows a long section on alternative methods of treatment including diet, supplements, herbs, and so on.

Although I explain carefully how candling works and provide fact sheets for all new patients, there are still some who get the idea that three candle treatments are all they need to do to cure anything, even a stubborn problem they have had for years. We are so used to quick solutions that it requires a whole new mindset to understand that health problems aren't solved in a flash. For some people that might be the case, but we are not all alike.

It does appear that illness frequently starts in our minds or emotions before it is evident in the body. Therefore, it follows that tracking back to what was going on when the illness first appeared can be extremely fruitful. Internationally recognized psychopharmacologist Candace Pert makes the following statement in her best-selling book *Molecules of Emotion: The Science Behind Body-Mind Medicine* (Hay House, 1997):

> The notion that others can make us feel good or bad is untrue. Why we feel the way we feel is the result of the symphony of our own molecules of emotion that affect every aspect of our physiology, producing blissful good health or miserable disease.

It is very important to remember this when hearing (or anything else) is impaired. A clear illustration was given by a lady suffering from tinnitus, who called one day to see if the candles could help her. She lived alone with her handicapped daughter and the stress of looking after the girl without any respite wasn't helping her condition. At the end of the conversation, when I explained that the candles were unlikely to be of much use in her case, she exclaimed: 'I can't stand it when she screams!'

We talked about the idea of her 'manufacturing' a different sound to block the distressing screams, but I don't know if she was ever able to look at the situation from that angle. White noise is something that is introduced into the ear to counteract the sounds caused by tinnitus. It doesn't seem to me that swapping one noise for another is going to help much, but perhaps some people have benefited.

A health-food shop owner, who is also a practitioner, called one day. A customer had complained how, on using the candles, she had felt pain in one ear. He admitted being rather abrupt with her, then he used the candles himself and found the same thing happened. When he spoke to me, he explained that it was his left side, and when asked if there was any current challenge with his mother, as traditionally that side of the body is associated with the feminine aspect, he replied that he'd forgotten that, and in fact had recently been dreaming of her constantly.

It is interesting that in the years since that conversation, I have come across quite a few middle-aged women with tinnitus in the left ear and, without exception, they have told me of a difficult relationship with their mothers.

Dr Christine Page, a doctor of medicine and a well-known writer on the connection between mind, body, and spirit, mentions in her book *The Mirror of Existence* (C.W. Daniel, 1996) that tinnitus relates to people not listening to their intuition. They prefer to continue asking everyone else's opinion until they receive an answer that resonates with their desire for minimal disruption in their lives and little personal responsibility, thus limiting any errors they may make.

An excellent book on psychosomatic illness with a section on ear problems is *The Healing Power of Illness* by Thorwald Dethlefson and Rudiger Dahlke (Element Books Ltd, 1983). The questions they ask at the end of the section on ears are related to why we may not be prepared to 'lend an ear' to other people, or what we may be refusing to hear.

Vertigo and Ménière's Disease

Ménière's disease is a condition affecting the inner ear (the labyrinth), which is comprised of tiny fluid-filled channels that help to transmit sound vibrations to the brain. Problems arise when the fluid builds up, causing the tissue to swell and affecting hearing and balance, which is also controlled by the labyrinth. Symptoms include vertigo and nausea. Sufferers frequently have perforated ear drums that never close up, so cranial osteopathy is worth a try here—it could even have a positive effect on the illness itself.

I have often been asked whether the candles could work for vertigo and Ménière's disease. One early customer did give me a testimonial saying that she was 'exceedingly delighted with the effect this [the candle treatment] is having on my vertigo/ear problems'.

I should have looked further into it with her, but at the time I had little experience.

A customer in New Zealand told me of the success she had had treating a man suffering from this unpleasant ailment. She was seeing him every week; one week ear candling and the next using head massage. Having learnt the pressure points to work on at home, her patient found that he was suffering fewer attacks, which were less severe and his hearing had improved.

In *The Complete Book of Water Therapy* (Contemporary Books, 2002), Dian Dincin Buchman suggests treating Ménière's disease by consuming foods that reduce water retention. Salt intake should be minimal, and she also suggests that an ear, nose, and throat practitioner should be consulted to see whether there are nasal polyps present.

Psychosomatic Links

The link between illness and the mind is becoming mainstream thinking. It is being explored in different ways all the time, and I find it utterly fascinating. It does appear that illness frequently starts in our minds or emotions before it is evident in the body.

It can be a lengthy and even painful process digging back to find the source of our health problems. We can weigh up every possibility, but it will pay dividends because when we touch on the very crux of the matter something in us *knows* instinctively that we've found the right answer, and only then can we go forward and do something about it.

A fascinating example of a psychosomatic cause for tinnitus was brought to my notice in an article in *Le Matin*, a Swiss newspaper, in 2003 about a Catholic priest who had always known of his homosexuality but, until he was ordained at the age of 32, had attempted to deny it. Thereafter, he had fought it and plunged into a nervous breakdown. Once again he endeavoured to hide his longings; until several months before he 'came out'. He described starting to experience a loud whistling sound in his left ear, which he interpreted as his soul crying out to speak its truth. The physical suffering was intense, and he decided to inform his bishop that he was leaving Holy Orders. The decision made, his tinnitus immediately calmed down and at the time the article appeared, he was practically cured.

One case of deafness concerned a man I knew personally who went stone deaf in his 40s. It just so happened that his wife never seemed to stop talking. She told me that she had even had to be hospitalized on one occasion due to difficulty in drawing breath. I'm not saying that her husband's deafness was 100 per cent due to her non-stop talking, but I feel it was a strong factor.

People with poor lymphatic circulation may be holding on to something and 'not going with the flow', according to Robyn Elizabeth Welch, a medical intuitive who describes how she works in her book *Conversations with the Body* (Hodder & Stoughton, 2002). She has found that people with rigid personalities not only have poor lymphatic flow but also kidney problems—again that kidneys/ears connection. In her opinion, their attitude to life makes them hang on to the inside of their bodies and this tightens the structure of the tissues.

CHAPTER 3

The Immune System: Vaccines, Allergies, and Nutrition

Because the main benefit of candling is its positive effect on the immune system, this book would not be complete without a little more information on this wonderful system and what it does.

So how does it work? Let me reiterate the information I gave at the beginning of the book, as it is really important to grasp this. Our whole body is irrigated by a liquid called lymph, which flows through a chain of capillaries, a system of tiny thread-like channels just below the skin. A series of lymphatic ganglions in strategic places, such as behind the ears, under the arms, in the groin, behind the knees and so on, receives this liquid from the capillaries and cleanses it of its impurities. When the lymph is flowing properly, our body is well protected against invaders.

Unlike the heart, which pumps the blood, there is no pump to send the lymph around the body, so it is through physical activity that it functions. We can avoid overloading our immune system by adopting a healthy lifestyle. Its job is to protect us from illness, and it is highly susceptible to suggestion. There is much evidence that meditation leads to better health and negative thoughts can have a negative effect on our bodies as well as our minds.

One major factor attacking the immune system was brought to my notice through a letter in a Swiss newspaper. Honorary Professor Yves Primault at the International University of Milan writing in *La Tribune de Genève* in 2000, reports that the secretion of melatonin, the hormone that regulates the sleep cycle, by the pineal gland in the brain is of primary importance to the immune system. His tells us that his studies have proved that when this gland is subjected to a field of 100 nanoTesla it ceases to produce melatonin. This can be caused by a radio-alarm clock beside the head of the bed and, what is more alarming, he found that one minute on a mobile phone can inhibit the secretion of melatonin for a week.

At the moment of birth, the immune system of a baby will be in perfect order if its mother has been treating her body well and preparing for her pregnancy. If she breastfeeds, the baby will benefit from the immune-enhancing proteins and amino acids contained in her breast milk. If she finds breastfeeding difficult, pumping the milk and putting it into bottles has proved to be the solution for some mothers—when the baby is put to the breast the amount taken at each feed can't be measured. A recent study has confirmed that breast milk helps a baby's brain to grow, and the duration of breastfeeding is positively associated with behavioural performance (Deoni, S.C., Dean, D.C. 3rd, Piryatinsky I., et al., 2013).[19] Colostrum, also known as first milk, which is present in the mammary glands just prior to birth, continues to be secreted in breast milk for the first few days. This is essential for the development of the baby's immune system, populating the gut with good and bad bacteria so that the system can learn to differentiate. This means that for the rest of the child's life the body will recognize and repel an invader. The immune system is fragile in a new-born and to ensure a healthy life, it needs to continue to develop without any aggression from outside for at least two years.

The first assault on the baby's system is when it is vaccinated. Vaccines are generally bound with adjuvants such as thimerosal (a derivative of mercury), viruses, formaldehyde, aluminium sulphate, and ammonium sulphate to keep them active. Aluminium is considered a developmental neurotoxin, with the ability to cross over the blood-brain barrier, getting stuck inside the brain. Its build-up over time can lead to Alzheimer's disease and central nervous system disorders.

David Christopher is a Master Herbalist and director of The School of Natural Healing in Springville, Utah. He is also a well-known broadcaster and popular international teacher and lecturer.

He has this to say about vaccinating infants: 'My main concern with vaccines is why do they inject them into babies? There is no immune memory til the child's immune system develops in the timeframe of 6 months to 18 months! No benefit, thousands of casualties. I am personally contacted by many women with children who were perfectly normal until these children received vaccines.'

Flu vaccines are recommended for babies, starting in the first few months, as well as for adults of all ages. The FDA in the United States has approved Flublok, a flu vaccine containing genetically modified proteins derived from insect cells. It is produced by extracting cells from a type of caterpillar and genetically altering them to produce large amounts of haemagglutinin, a flu virus protein that enables the flu virus itself to enter the body quickly. The manufacturers admit that two study participants died during the trials, but they still insist that Flublok is safe! One of the possible side effects they mention is the nerve virus Guillain-Barré Syndrome, which has been shown to be a side effect of other flu vaccines.

Another side effect of giving the flu vaccine to children, reported at the 105th International Conference of the American Thoracic Society, was that vaccinated children were three times more likely to need hospital care than children who had not received the vaccine, with asthmatic children being especially vulnerable. The Mayo Clinic in Rochester made the discovery after studying 263 children who had had flu and whether or not they had been vaccinated.

There have been many studies carried out and much evidence collected on people who weren't vaccinated against childhood illnesses and who caught all of them. As adults, their immune systems have proved healthier than those who were vaccinated, as the fevers associated with these illnesses burn off the impurities and strengthen the person's immunity. They also seem to be less prone to develop cancer in later life. It is interesting to note that children who suffer from ailments such as mumps or measles never contract the same illnesses again, as they have built up their immunity to them. Parents often report that a 'growth spurt' has followed recovery from a childhood illness; when the body is about to undertake a major change, the immune system becomes stressed.

Years ago, when children developed a routine ailment, the mother would organize a party for their playmates to be exposed to it, and thereby get over it while it was still at a low level of inconvenience. Much better than to catch the illness in adulthood, as I can attest, passing on the mumps I developed as a child to my mother, who had a much more painful experience.

In addition, most doctors, not having a knowledge of traditional Chinese medicine, can easily inject into a meridian line and cause it to block. According to a naturopathic practitioner, as the energy flow becomes more and more sluggish through that meridian, health problems can appear many years later. In fact, as many vaccines are relatively new, we have no idea about their long-term effects throughout a person's life. Now that more and more vaccines are being injected at the same time, there is no history of the synergy of these vaccines and whether they should all be given in one shot. Nothing synthetic, such as vaccines and allopathic drugs, comes 'free'—the side effects can appear much farther down the road, when everyone has forgotten the one thing that could have caused them.

There has been much discussion about the connection between multiple vaccines and autism. Dr Andrew Wakefield, a gastroenterologist who first drew attention to this possible link, was vilified and his licence to practice in the UK withdrawn when he found that autistic children were missing three vital bacteria in their gut and surmised that the measles, mumps, and rubella (MMR) vaccine could be the reason. Researchers at Arizona State University have validated his findings on the lower levels of gut bacteria, although they have not at the time of writing discovered why. Their full report was published in *PLOS ONE,* a peer-reviewed journal, in July 2013 (Kang D-W., Park J.G., et al., 2013).[20] A video entitled *AutismOne & Generation Rescue 2013 Conference Congressional Panel,* which first appeared in May 2013, highlights the fact that in 1980, 1 in 10,000 children suffered from autism and in 2013, the figure had reduced to 1 in 50.[21] The expert witnesses from the Centers for Disease Control and Prevention (CDC) admitted that no research has ever been done to compare vaccinated against unvaccinated children to see whether it is the thimerosal in the vaccines that is causing the enormous rise in cases.

As so many of today's young mothers were vaccinated as children and have been treated with allopathic medicine throughout their lives, perhaps not always following a healthy diet, babies being born now are on average far less healthy than a couple of generations ago: all the more reason to take great care of a new-born and protect it from any treatments that could cause lasting damage.

It has been found that children living in the isolated Amish community in the United States, which eschews many modern practices, do not experience the problems of autism and learning difficulties found in the general population. They eat healthy organic food, which is home grown, and the children are unvaccinated. Even among adults, heart disease, diabetes and cancer are relatively unknown. The simple and healthy Amish lifestyle should be proof to all of us that we are responsible for our health. The simpler we keep things, the healthier we are likely to be.

Vaccination does not always do what it is supposed to do, either, and for people who have already been vaccinated against any illness, it is also wise to have homoeopathic antidotes made up that remove some of its negative effects.

In 2010, a news story by Reuters reported that whooping cough outbreaks are higher among vaccinated children compared with unvaccinated children. According to the Reuters report, in early 2010, a spike in cases of whooping cough appeared at Kaiser Permanente Medical Center, the largest seen in California in more than 50 years. Dr David Witt, an infectious disease specialist at the medical center, was quoted as saying: 'We started dissecting the data. What was very surprising was that the majority of cases were in fully vaccinated children. That's what started catching our attention.'

Writing on *www.preventdisease.com*, Dave Mihalovic in 2012 quoted data from the Vermont Department of Health in the United States suggesting that going through the pertussis (whooping cough) vaccination regimen was not solving the problem or warding off this highly contagious disease. If anything, it appeared to be making it worse. A study in *The New England Journal of Medicine* (Klein,

N.P., Bartlett, J., et al., 2012)[22] showed that the vaccine was not effective after a certain period and many experts were speculating that its effectiveness was nil from the very first injection in the series.

An article on *www.setyoufreenews.com* reported that in 2012, Vigo County, Indiana, was in the grip of an epidemic of chicken pox. It was stated that out of the 97 cases reported at that moment only three had never been vaccinated.

Over 30 years ago, I worked with the father of a small boy who was given a booster vaccine (I don't remember which one) while suffering from a slight cold. The doctor didn't consider this a problem, but within hours the child's body was burning up with fever and, had his parents not been lucky enough to live next door to a nurse with quick reflexes, it is unlikely he would have survived. And this was before the era of multiple vaccines.

If you are thinking about becoming pregnant and vaccinating your child or being vaccinated yourself, you might find it instructive to watch *Shots in the Dark*, a Canadian documentary that is completely free to view online on YouTube. You could also check out what Dr Vernon Coleman has to say about vaccines and many other health issues on his website: *www.vernoncoleman.com*. An informed choice makes for a better choice.

Another element that alters a baby's immune system is the administration of synthetic antibiotics, which destroy both good and bad intestinal bacteria and, because certain neuro-chemicals are manufactured in the gut, the baby's neurology is also altered. When all the bacteria have been destroyed in this way, the immune system's ability to manufacture the appropriate immunity-boosting cells is unlikely to recover fully.

This applies to adults, too, and just one course of antibiotics will effect a change. Many years of appropriate nutrition and probiotic treatment are then required to try and bring the body back to a reasonable level of health.

After an operation or a course of allopathic drugs, it is a good idea to note the names of the products used and a homoeopathic chemist will make up antidotes to flush them from the system. I did this after an operation to mend a broken wrist, but during a colonic irrigation two months later, the therapist found that there were still chemical residues left in the gut.

Allergies, which offer evidence of a compromised immune system, frequently affect the nose and sinuses, and they tend to be set off by exposure to dust, pollen, mould, chemicals, and food. Patrick Holford and Dr James Brialy, in *Hidden Food Allergies* (Piatkus, 2006) consider one of the major offenders to be cow's milk, and they give the following list of how it can affect children and adults: middle ear infections, poor sleep patterns, eczema, migraines, rheumatoid arthritis, hyperactivity, bronchitis, frequent infections, non-seasonal allergic rhinitis, bedwetting in children, colic, heartburn, indigestion, chronic diarrhoea, chronic fatigue syndrome, hypersensitivity, depression, autism, and possibly type 1 diabetes. Which is really a pretty impressive list! An allergy to cow's milk can contribute to iron deficiency, as it blocks the absorption of iron, and this can lead to anaemia.

Other well-known offenders are soy products, yeast, wheat, eggs, chocolate, citrus, and beans, although when beans are eaten frequently as part of a balanced diet by vegetarians they cause fewer problems. Vaccines are often cultured on hen's eggs, which is why many children are allergic to eggs. For people who are allergic to soy products, careful inspection of labels is called for, as many, many foodstuffs contain soy; most commercially marketed margarines are made from soy oil, as noted earlier. As mentioned in the section Children and Candles, testing for food allergies will rapidly show which foodstuffs we need to eliminate

A homoeopathic doctor explained during a conference I attended that the huge increase in people suffering from allergies in their thirties and forties is a direct result of the vaccines they received as children, although I have found no other evidence either to confirm or deny this. Several studies have shown that vaccinated children often go on to develop the illness against which they were vaccinated later in life (if not whilst they are still young, as we have seen above) and when they do, it is usually a stronger variant.

Allergies to animal dander are common. One man in the UK, who had grown up with dogs in the family, was plagued with what he thought was hay fever from the age of seven. It was only when he and his wife decided to get two dogs themselves that he started suffering very badly, and a skin prick test revealed that he was allergic to his dogs. Candling is a great help in treating allergies and could even cure the root cause.

Echinacea is a terrific immune system booster, as mentioned earlier, and homoeopathy also works very well for many complaints, certainly for allergies: the bonus it offers is that it has no known side effects.

Many of the problems children experience with their ears come from an excess of sugar, as touched on in the last chapter. It is, therefore, important to ensure that from the moment they start on solids, children are given foods that don't contain sugar, and certainly not artificial sweeteners. An excellent replacement (although in strict moderation) is stevia, which comes from a plant native to Paraguay and which has been used for centuries. Sweeter than sugar, it is even suitable for diabetics and contains absolutely no calories. Unfortunately, it can have a slight aftertaste.

Xylitol is a natural sugar that comes from birch bark. Our bodies also produce up to 15 grams of xylitol from other food sources, and it is widely distributed throughout nature in small amounts. Some of the best sources are fruits, berries, mushrooms, lettuce, and corn cobs. One cup of raspberries contains almost one gram of xylitol. There are synthetic forms of xylitol on the market and it is vitally important to find a natural product. It appears to be becoming more popular as I see it in all the health food shops in my city. (See also Chapter 2: Children and Candles.)

It is never a good idea to let children develop a taste for sweetening or salting foods, as they inevitably mask the real taste of the ingredients. An excess of either may not only lead to problems in later life but also mean that their meals will need to be loaded with one or the other to appeal to their palates.

The homoeopath I mentioned earlier who gave the mother a list of the foods to be avoided by her son with ear problems seems very logical. Dietary measures should be the first line of treatment in situations like this. It would save a great deal of time and money if, instead of immediately doling out drugs or signing patients up for expensive examinations, doctors looked first into lifestyle issues; nutrition and state of mind play a huge part in how we heal or whether we fall ill. That is not to say that we are not responsible for our health; we need to be proactive, and there is plenty of valuable information out there if we care to look for it.

Another problem for the immune system that has come to the fore is the danger from genetically modified organisms (GMOs). The reason so many people have an allergy to wheat products is thought to be due to the genetic modifications that have taken place in wheat over the centuries; this is why spelt—a very ancient form of wheat—is better digested. In *Seeds of Deception* (Green Books, 1994), his devastating exposé of the biotechnology industry, Jeffrey M. Smith explains how disastrous GMOs have proved to be and how information on the illnesses and, in some instances, deaths caused by their use, has been suppressed and any trial pointing in that direction immediately halted.

Glyphosate, which is an ingredient of Monsanto's Roundup® herbicide, is extremely toxic, and a body of evidence is accumulating on the National Library of Medicines MEDLINE database (*www.medline.com*) showing that glyphosate-based agri-chemicals have been linked to over 40 health conditions from Parkinson's disease to leukaemia. Glyphosate has also been implicated in over two dozen modes of toxicity, from causing damage to DNA and disrupting hormone receptors to suppressing the immune system and damaging neurons.

Also, more and more countries are refusing to plant Monsanto's genetically modified wheat and corn, and there has been huge resistance worldwide. With some countries now also refusing to import genetically modified wheat from the United States, this could lead to some interesting developments. In India, hundreds of thousands of small farmers have already joined together to reject genetically modified seeds. In some places, laws have been passed requiring products containing genetically modified organisms (GMOs) to be clearly labelled; a movement is growing in the United States, in particular, to compel food manufacturers, health food stores, and groceries to label such foods; many companies have now signed on to have their products independently certified as free of GMOs by the Non-GMO Project. With so many countries now refusing these products, and pressure being put on manufacturers to label their products clearly so that consumers can see what they are buying, there is hope for the future.

A class action suit by five million soybean farmers was brought against Monsanto in Brazil in 2012. Brazil is a country that has gone in for massive GMO production, but the plaintiffs have benefited from a court ruling that it is illegal to demand annual royalties of 2 per cent on 'renewal' crops—seeds that have been saved from previous years—an impossible financial burden for small farms. Monsanto lost the case on appeal and was ordered to pay US$ 7.5 billion in compensation.

It is also well to bear in mind that much of what we eat has been treated with all kinds of different chemicals. Although in some places the choice of organic food may be restricted and is sometimes more expensive, it is a good investment and it certainly ensures that we eat more locally grown fruit and vegetables when they are in season. People who have allergies to kiwi fruit, say, have often discovered that, through eating organic varieties, they're not allergic to the fruit itself but to the pesticides. Similarly for wine drinkers who experience headaches after a glass of wine, organic wine can be the solution. For meat and fish, too, it is important to eat organic. A colleague, whose brother farmed in Scotland, told me many years ago that his family had stopped eating meat because he realized how often the vet was being called in to treat his animals. When we eat animals that have been treated with antibiotics we are obviously consuming the latter at the same time and building up our resistance so that, in a case of emergency, they can be ineffective.

Non-organic fish farms have a very poor reputation for heavy pollution of the surrounding seas. Salmon are fed pellets made from ground-up fish and oils, and the fish used for these usually come from the seabed, where the polluted run-off from rivers accumulates, making them highly toxic. Antibiotics in vast quantities are also needed for farmed fish to prevent them from getting diseases that make them inedible. Salmon used to be a fish that only wealthy people could afford; now it is among the cheapest, due to the growth in fish farming. This fact alone should ring alarm bells.

An anti-abortion group in the US, Children of God for Life, has called on the public to boycott products from major food and beverage companies that collaborate with a biotech company producing flavour enhancers: the biotech company uses tissue from aborted foetuses in testing, and the anti-abortion group is in favour of using animal cells, instead. Aside from the moral question of using either, it is repellent that not only does the flavour of these products need to be enhanced but that a biotech company is doing the work. The company states rather disingenuously that manufacturers want to reduce monosodium glutamate (MSG), sugar, and salt in their foods and this is an excellent solution. Our cells are living organisms, and if we eat and drink chemicals it is inevitable that they have to work harder to process these foreign bodies and will likely break down sooner.

Dr Vernon Coleman, in his book *Food for Thought* (The European Journal Publishing House, 1994), reports that a growing number of doctors have noticed that asthma, dermatitis, eczema, hay fever and rhinitis seem to predominate in people who eat a lot of junk food (inevitably loaded with additives of every type, usually cheap ones to keep costs down) or dairy produce, and that a change of diet would be extremely beneficial.

Still on the subject of nutrition, there has been a most interesting development in Russia, and that's the allocation of plots of land to ordinary folk as a result of a decree in 2003 by then President Vladimir Putin. Every Russian citizen has the right to a plot in perpetuity on which to construct a small dwelling and to plant fruit and vegetables and keep chickens or a goat or two. Although plots were initially granted on poor soil, a huge network of eco-villages has developed, with the bulk of Russia's fruit, vegetables, meat and milk supplied by these amazingly fertile and successful projects without the use of chemicals or GMOs.

This means that the majority of Russians must be eating organic food without having to search it out or pay more for it! The idea has now spread round the world, and the thousands of small villages that have sprung up celebrate Gardeners' Day on 23 July each year. It is well worth a mention here, where we're discussing allergy-causing GMOs and how to overcome their negative effect. If all those people round the world who have the possibility of producing fruit, vegetables, eggs, and so forth for sale manage to do it even on a small scale, they will vastly raise awareness of the importance of fresh, organic food and the improved taste.

I mentioned the artificial sweetener aspartame earlier in connection with tinnitus; it is also included in most chewing gums. As with anything held and chewed in the mouth, gum goes rapidly into the bloodstream. What is perhaps even more alarming is that it also contains maltitol, mannitol, and sorbitol, sugar alcohols used in a vast number of 'low-sugar' products that have been shown to cause abdominal pains and diarrhoea, whilst aggravating various health conditions, such as irritable bowel syndrome. Therefore, exposure to them is going to hit the immune system hard. In fact, a look at the contents of the commercially marketed chewing gums will show them to be a cocktail of chemicals and better left alone. There is much more information on this on *www.healthwyze.org*, a highly informative website with articles on a quantity of health-related matters. Gum from health food shops will only contain healthy ingredients and is usually sweetened with xylitol. (See Chapter 2, Children and Candles.)

It is now possible to buy non-toxic paints that do not contain volatile organic compounds (VOC), for use indoors and out. There are also curtains on the market that cut out the electromagnetic field (EMF) pollution suffered by people who live on main roads, next to railway junctions, or opposite mobile phone masts. They are not cheap, but tests with professional EMF meters have shown them to be very effective. There are also various devices that may be purchased to protect us against the effects of this pollution.

In his book *Domestic Medicine*, first published in 1785, Dr William Buchan wrote that too much reliance was being placed on medicines and not enough on a healthy lifestyle. (An online version can be found on *http://www.americanrevolution.org/medicine.html*.)

This is what he says: 'The man who pays proper attention to [diet, air, exercise, and the natural healing capacity of the human body] will seldom need the physician, and he who does not will seldom enjoy health. . .' I couldn't agree more: the immune system thrives on a healthy diet, proper exercise, and sufficient sleep, together with a positive outlook on life, and if we listen to and act on the messages our bodies send us, there is no reason why we shouldn't live to a very happy, healthy, and active old age.

Ototoxic Medication

Allopathic drugs can cause hearing problems, notably hearing loss and tinnitus, which greatly diminish our enjoyment of life, according to new information. Many of these drugs are available over the counter, but it isn't advisable to take anything that can result in side effects without consulting a specialist.

A very useful article in *Alternatif Bien-Être*, a Swiss magazine for holistic practitioners, gives details of the kinds of allopathic medication to avoid. In fact, since 2008, more than 130 drugs feature on the list. I've taken a few examples from the article, which is based on a study published in the *American Journal of Medicine* in 2010 (Curhan, S.C., Eavey, R., et al., 2010).[23]

Researchers found that, taken over long periods, NSAIDS (non-steroidal anti-inflammatory drugs) such as aspirin, acetaminophen (Paracetamol), and ibuprofen (Nurofen) appear to affect the hearing of men more than any other section of the population—the younger the men, the more damage they cause. Paracetamol has proved especially toxic, affecting hearing in 99 per cent of regular users under the age of 50 as opposed to 61 per cent of habitual users of non-corticoid anti-inflammatories and 33 per cent of regular users of aspirin.

I have known since I started working with the candles that aspirin (salicylic acid) affects the kidneys, and I have met many people, especially at health exhibitions, who tell me they take aspirin as a blood thinner and also suffer from tinnitus. As mentioned earlier, according to traditional Chinese medicine (TCM), the kidneys and ears are located on the same meridian line in the body, so sufferers may be helped by finding a replacement for aspirin.

People with a headache, a fever, or a pain somewhere are often inclined to take an aspirin or two, but it cannot be emphasized strongly enough that just because it's sold over the counter, aspirin is by no means something that can be swallowed without risk. It is a powerful drug and, dulling the body's cry for attention (which is the role of pains and fevers), is no solution and can make matters worse, as the underlying cause has not been treated.

Another drug likely to have a deleterious effect on hearing is codeine, when it is used over long periods. **NOTE:** the UK Medicines and Healthcare Products Regulatory Agency (MHRA) has issued an alert to doctors in the UK to stop prescribing codeine to under-12s, following the reported deaths of several children who had been given it. It is also an active ingredient in children's cough medicines, so care must be taken with these. Migraine sufferers who have come to rely on codeine during attacks find in the long run that it worsens the condition, and unfortunately it can become addictive: other solutions must be found.

According to the study mentioned above, hearing problems can also be caused by certain diuretics, and some antibiotics have been known to cause tinnitus. I treated a patient who had been taking antibiotics and who was left with slight tinnitus. She knew about ear candles, and after three treatments she had no further problem. She comes to me every now and then, when she finds a cold hard to shake off or when she feels the need.

Some of the medication used in the treatment of cancer has been seen to cause ear problems, and another element that I found interesting was the case of antimalarial medication. A patient suffering from tinnitus consulted me several years ago. Her problem could have been compounded from being hit in the face when she was young, as nothing had been done at the time to see whether any long-term damage had been sustained. We cleared the tinnitus with ear candle treatments and she was delighted. However, shortly afterwards she went to Africa on holiday and took chloroquine (a prophylactic against malaria) which is advised for travellers to areas where malaria is endemic. Once she was back home the tinnitus returned and as she lived miles away, we lost touch. However, reading in this study that chloroquine can cause ear problems, I feel that is exactly what could have happened.

Lynne McTaggart, the award-winning journalist who is joint editor of the newsletter *What Doctors Don't Tell You,* writes that in the United States, a quarter of the prescriptions for antibiotics are for children with ear problems, although it has been seen that a wait-and-see approach is often a better first step. Despite this heavy dosing with antibiotics, incidences of middle ear infection have soared. I do understand that many people who consult a doctor will insist on receiving a prescription for antibiotics, as they feel they have not been taken seriously if they don't come out clutching one; as a result, the doctor often buckles under the pressure.

In cases where an antibiotic may be necessary, and where the patient's life is at risk, obviously quick action is vital. McTaggart reports, however, that doctors tend to prescribe an antibiotic *before* lab tests have shown what the problem is and the patient might be half-way through the course when the doctor realizes that the antibiotic prescribed wasn't suitable for that particular pathology. She further reports that children who have taken more than 20 courses of antibiotics between the ages of one and 12 are more likely to suffer from developmental problems, as well as ear infections, than children who have received three or fewer doses of antibiotics throughout the same period. McTaggart mentions that heavy antibiotic use in children can affect their hearing, and overuse in the developing world (where some antibiotics are sold over the counter) has caused an epidemic of deafness.

Never flush unwanted antibiotics down the lavatory or put them in the garbage as they go into landfill and seep out into the environment. Creams, ointments, and soaps can contain antibacterial agents, and these obviously build up our resistance to antibiotics, making them less effective if we do need them. One of the best ways to ensure good health is to practise good hygiene, washing our hands regularly, certainly when coming in from outside, after visits to the lavatory and before preparing food.

If for any reason you have been prescribed a course of antibiotics by your doctor, it must always be followed to the end, as stopping it too soon can cause the infection to gain strength and become resistant to further treatment.

CHAPTER 4

Where Something
Else Is Needed

Cranial Osteopathy – Craniosacral Therapy

Greg Webb, RMP, (see Chapter 5) tells us that ear candling has been found to enhance cranial bone articulation, as well as the circulation of the cerebrospinal fluid (CSF) around the brain and spinal cord, which is essential to health in the body. It is important to note, though, that many candle treatments may be required, and certain conditions cannot be greatly improved by using ear candles. In such cases, I recommend cranial osteopathy, otherwise known as craniosacral therapy, a century-old treatment that works at a very deep level to improve cerebrospinal fluid flow in the craniosacral system and well-being throughout the whole body.

Cases where craniosacral therapy can be helpful include situations where the body has been subject to some kind of physical damage, such as a blow to the head, exposure to loud noise, or an eardrum perforation that never closes. This is also why many rock musicians (past and present) suffer from constant noise in the ears. People who work with machines or on building sites, sound engineers, who spend all day with earphones clamped to their ears, and people who frequent discothèques or places where very loud music is played, are invariably affected. It was also suggested to a friend whose baby had a difficult birth that two or three sessions with a cranial osteopath would be advisable, and he loved it.

In *Spontaneous Healing* (Sphere, 1996), Dr Andrew Weil writes about cranial osteopath Dr Robert Fulford of Tucson, Arizona, now deceased, who had great success in treating children, particularly those with 'glue ear'. He relates that in only one craniosacral session, during which Dr Fulford concentrated on freeing up restrictions in the sacrum blocking cerebrospinal fluid circulation, he had been able to cure the condition. His theory in this case was that the sacral end of the craniosacral system is frequently 'locked up' in children, probably from birth trauma. He continues quoting Dr Fulford by adding that, according to the latter, when there are restrictions in the sacrum, it leads to impairment of the primary respiratory mechanism, the subtle 'breath' beneath the regular breath that allows health-giving cerebrospinal fluid to circulate throughout the central nervous system.

Once the cerebrospinal fluid is able to flow unimpeded throughout the craniosacral system, the other systems of the body start to come online again, and health is restored from the inside out, starting with the nervous system, which sends messages throughout the body about how to maintain health. In the case of 'glue ear', on the physical level, poor fluid drainage from the head and neck due to restrictions in the bones and tissues leads to a situation where stagnant fluid builds up in the middle ear. Once the craniosacral system has been restored to healthy functioning, the body's own self-healing mechanism takes over and drainage naturally occurs.

A lady came to consult me at a health exhibition, asking if the candles could help with her tinnitus. I asked her when it had started and if she knew what had caused it. She said that about a year before, a heavy dish had fallen on her head and, although she had asked her doctor if there was any connection, he had assured her that there was none. We explained that she could well have dislocated one or more of the tiny bones in the middle ear, or even a cervical vertebra, and that cranial osteopathy would be the most likely avenue to explore for help.

A similar experience occurred a few years ago, when a young man also suffering from tinnitus asked the same question. We talked for a long while and, during the course of the conversation, he mentioned that he had injured his shoulder playing rugby at school. As the tinnitus was confined to one ear, the obvious question was whether it was on the same side of the body. When he confirmed that it was, it became clear that cranial osteopathy would be a good option to try to clear the tinnitus and his old shoulder injury.

I was consulted by a lady about tinnitus that had developed in one of her ears. She felt that it had come on after watching some noisy floats going past at an annual parade, all blaring out hard rock-type music. I suggested she try cranial osteopathy, as the noise vibration had likely been responsible for her problem and candles would not be the solution.

Being subjected to constant noise is a great challenge for people who live in cities. Children are now being assailed by levels of noise that are more than likely to lead to problems in later years. In fact the organisers of the event mentioned above provide ear plugs for them if they are coming to watch the parade.

Another therapy strongly recommended for headaches, migraines, tinnitus, and possibly sinusitis is AtlasPROfilax (*www.atlasprofilax.com*). This treatment consists of gently pushing the atlas, which is the first cervical vertebra, back into its correct position. The atlas is out of place in just about everybody, and only one session is needed to correct this with a follow-up to check. Something I found extremely interesting was that children born to mothers whose atlas had been correctly aligned were also born with theirs in place. With such a delicate treatment it is, of course, essential to consult a practitioner who has been trained and has qualified in the method taught by the academy set up by René-Claudius Schümperli, the founder, and qualified AtlasProf®s can be found in over 30 countries.

My personal experience of this therapy was that it increased the mobility in my neck. Initially, I was able to turn my head much farther one side than the other, and after a simple treatment I had the same degree of mobility on both sides. A Swiss journalist, Francis Georges Perrin, decided to investigate before undergoing the treatment himself. His book, *La correction de l'atlas* (Editions à la Carte, 2006) is chock full of accounts by people who had suffered from numerous health problems and who found relief through this method. I read his book before trying it out and it easily convinced me.

Clay Therapy

This is a well-known treatment in continental Europe, and there are many books on the subject. Clay is quite amazing—a clay poultice will draw out toxins and will even turn a baby improperly placed in the womb. Its bio-mineral composition acts differently on each person and each problem it encounters. The body absorbs the minerals it needs from the clay, using them to help heal, balance, and restore vitality. At the same time, the clay absorbs impurities from the system. After use, it must be disposed of very carefully, as just casually dumping it in the garden will kill every living thing around it.

For ear problems, treatment invariably consists of clay poultices behind the ear and around the nape of the neck (having first placed a small cotton wool plug in each ear to protect it). The pioneer of clay healing was Raymond Dextreit, whose seminal book *L'argile qui guérit* is still available in its original language although its first edition dates back over 40 years. It was translated into English as *Our Earth, Our Cure* (Citadel Press, 1993) by Michel Abehsera who was much inspired by Dextreit's work and who wrote *The Healing Clay* (Citadel Press, 1979) with loads of useful information on the external uses of clay. In it, he suggested cleansing the colon and using clay poultices on the lower abdomen, as this can be highly beneficial in the case of ear infections, too. These two books are now out of print, although one of Abehsera's books still available is *The Healing Power of Clay: The Natural Remedy for Dozens of Common Ailments* (Citadel Press, 2001).

Using clay internally is comprehensively covered in *The Clay Cure* (Healing Arts Press, 1998) by Ran Knishinsky. He has been 'eating dirt', as he terms it, for many years and has acquired a wealth of experience on the different types of clay and the effects of taking it internally.

Knishinsky reports that clay can be used to treat a variety of health problems, including diarrhoea, constipation, and acne. He tells us that his brother cleared a case of acne within one week of taking clay and, combined with the candles and an appropriate diet, it must be a very powerful way of dealing with this unpleasant and unsightly problem. He also finds it suitable for allergies, where the liver becomes saturated with toxins and fatty tissue, making it unable to produce the antihistamines necessary to combat hay fever and other allergies.

As already mentioned, I have had great success in treating allergies just using the candles—lasting success, in fact, as several patients who have had two or three treatments find their sensitivity to allergens has completely disappeared and they sail through the seasons with no difficulty.

The benefit of taking clay internally was confirmed by a friend. She was prescribed antibiotics by an allopathic practitioner and suffered from intestinal burning, which can arise after a long period on antibiotics. She decided to try taking clay internally to soothe the discomfort and found it helped greatly.

Similarly, the husband of another friend, also taking a long course of synthetic antibiotics, was able to calm his irritated gut, although he was unfortunately against the idea of trying to find an alternative treatment for his initial problem.

Another great use of clay is to reduce swelling, although swelling usually means that the body is protecting itself from some internal hurt and that should be investigated first. It is a bit messy, but, once the paste has been applied, a layer of cling film to seal it will not only keep the clay moist but ensure that it doesn't smear itself over everything else.

Whichever way clay is used, it is a very powerful healing tool and one that it is worth investigating.

Manual Lymph Drainage

I became interested in the Vodder method of manual lymph drainage (MLD) in the treatment of tinnitus when I read an article by Michel Bontemps, a well-known local therapist, in a Swiss newspaper, *Genève Home Informations,* in October 2003, where he pronounced it his method of choice for dealing with this condition. MLD works on the underlying causes of illness, improving the circulation and rebalancing the central nervous system, with the latter enabling the vertebrae to realign spontaneously. He also suggested the use of specific herbs and a visit to an osteopath to check on the alignment of the vertebrae.

Few patients think of tinnitus and lymphatic drainage in the same breath, but having taken an introductory course in this gentle technique, I believe it could be beneficial. Dr Emil Vodder discovered it in the 1930s, while he was working in the South of France with a British patient who spent his winters there as he suffered so badly from sinusitis in the damp English climate. Unable to relieve the patient's symptoms any other way, Dr Vodder devised a method of pushing the lymph gently along the sinuses with the tips of his fingers, draining it into the lymphatic ganglions behind the ear.

It is important to find a practitioner who has learnt and understood the Vodder method, as there are therapists who purport to practise it but are either not being honest or have not grasped the basic principles. Lymph flows just below the skin and requires motion to move it along throughout the body. MLD is a relaxing, passive method of achieving the same thing (hence its name). The therapist uses the tips of the fingers and sometimes the palm of the hand in a gentle circular motion to 'pump' the lymph to be purified through the chain of lymphatic ganglions to facilitate the drainage process.

On my weekend course with Evelyne Selosse, who was trained by Dr Vodder, I learnt that the lymph capillaries are rather like pea pods and it takes only a light touch to push the lymph along to the next tiny cavity; a heavy touch blocks the flow, so that the 'peas' can't move.

I did an ear candle treatment on a patient who, after a bout with breast cancer seven years earlier, had been left with a slightly swollen arm that sometimes caused her discomfort. Some of the lymphatic ganglions in her armpit had been excised 'just in case', although they were found to be healthy. After the very first ear candle treatment, her arm became less swollen and more flexible as the lymph started to circulate properly.

There are several contraindications to lymphatic drainage, such as active cancer, acute inflammation, congestive heart failure, and blood clots, so do consult an experienced practitioner.

As far as tinnitus is concerned, and, as I have tried to show, it has multiple causes, this method on its own is unlikely to be successful in every case on a one-size-fits-all basis. In complementary medicine each patient is treated as an individual, so there cannot be one single remedy that works for everyone. When people are looking for ways to deal with the horrors of an affliction such as tinnitus they may, however, want to give it a try.

Fuller information on the function and benefits of manual lymphatic drainage for cancer treatment is included in the following chapter.

CHAPTER 5

Ear Candling and Cancer Therapy

*by Patrick Quanten, MD, (UK) and
Greg Webb, RMT, (Canada)*

Ear candling, an ancient ritual and healing art, which formed an integral part of cultures such as those of the Egyptians, Aztecs, and North American Indians, has found its way into our culture and into alternative medicine. Having 'rediscovered' it from the Native Americans, it has captured the imagination of many through its amazing effects and its simplicity. People all over the world are astonished at how different they feel when they have been 'candled'. And the growing interest, together with the absolute safety of the ear candling process itself, has allowed a great variety of people to be exposed to it. This in turn delivers many personal experiences and testimonies, including those suggesting that it is of great benefit to cancer sufferers.

But don't we hear that about every so-called 'new treatment'? Maybe so, but as regards ear candling, we can actually explain how and why it will improve your health, even when you are suffering from such a devastating disease.

But first, we will have to enlighten you on the disease process which leads to cancer. And you thought that nobody knows how someone gets cancer! Think again. It has been known for a long time; and at the same time it has been vehemently denied because accepting this knowledge would turn our whole medical culture bottom up. The process which leads to disease has been known to man since the dawn of time, long before cancer was 'invented'. How people get ill has not and cannot change throughout the ages, the only thing that changes is the expression of the disease. So what is this disease process which has been written up in ancient texts across the globe, surviving time and cultures?

The Disease Process

In spite of common belief, no disease happens quickly, no disease is acute; some expressions may be, but the process has to have been going on for quite some time before the medical profession recognizes it as a 'disease'. Naming and labelling is extremely important to doctors, it is part of their *prevention* strategy as well as their therapeutic approach. However, diseases are caused by a persistent imbalance within the system. Rather than naming the disease, it is about recognizing imbalances and correcting them before they damage the system and make us ill. Because all diseases are caused this way, it follows that essentially there are no 'new' diseases, only variations of the same basic disease-causing factors.

'Imbalance within the system'—meaning what exactly? Well, the system (body and mind) has an unbreakable contract to keep you well, fit, and healthy. It has a complete and accurate knowledge of every cellular function, every biochemical activity, and every aspect of our energy system. Every second it performs billions of actions without ever making a major mistake. (Fancy our computers doing that!) If a tiny thing is not entirely right it will recognize and rectify it straight away.

Trust your system to be 100 per cent committed to your health and well-being. It will do the very best that is possible, given the material it has been handed by you. And that is where most of the time the struggle starts! For the sake of simplicity we will consider this 'imbalance' as *any kind of deviation from 'the norm', or from what the system considers normal.*

This deviation, we call 'toxic'. A load of toxins puts the system out of balance; a prelude to ill-health. So, a toxin is by definition: *anything which, at that particular moment in time, the system does not need in order to maintain its health balance.* These toxins can enter the system from outside or can be entirely produced inside the system as part of the way it handles whatever life throws at it. Toxins, created internally as well as those entering the system from the outside, can be unnatural products that are alien to the system; they can be inappropriate or excessive items even though they are natural. Wrong timing and wrong combination of actions can also result in toxins.

These toxins now accumulate in the places where they have been collected and/or produced, mostly the digestive tract. They cause very few minor disturbances, such as very occasional distension, constipation, acidity, anger, indigestion, heaviness, or fatigue. As more and more toxins collect, the symptom pattern will increase both in frequency and severity. However, all the symptoms are vague and are quickly dismissed because 'everybody complains of those things and you just have to live with it'.

As the collection site is getting fuller an overflow will occur into other parts of the body, causing a different set of symptoms. Depending on the organs and tissues that are affected one can suffer from complaints such as dry skin, stiff joints, headaches, cough, constipation, lack of energy, swollen glands, fever, vomiting, dizzy spells, diarrhoea, tummy pains, etc. These symptoms occur more persistently, and doctors will now start to take notice. However, *all the medical tests will come back as normal.*

Those sites that are the weakest and most vulnerable will suffer the most. These particular locations will start to show signs of being unable to cope with the increasing amount of toxins coming their way. Symptoms will now be fixed in certain positions, corresponding with the troubled organ or tissues, and it is at this stage that *the doctor declares you have a particular disease,* such as asthma, diabetes, arthritis, cancer, or whatever it may happen to be. Finally, we can all be happy because they have found the problem. Congratulations, you have just graduated from hypochondriac to patient!

Further accumulation of toxins will induce a more widespread breakdown of tissues which is generally known as the disease complications.

Cancer

Cancer has many causes, as we all know, including our toxic environment, devitalized foods (produced and sold by the food industry), sedentary lifestyle (lack of appropriate exercise), and lack of spiritual purpose or effort in life. Its basis is often suppressed emotion or emotional stagnation, which causes accumulation of toxic material, the manifestation in physical (chemical) form of feelings. This was well known in the early days of western medicine, when cancer was described as a disease of melancholy, or 'black bile', which also translates as suppressed emotions. Hence, physical remedial measures are usually not enough to restore health, as our current track record in cancer treatment confirms.

The build-up of toxins happens because the digestive fire and other energy sources are low. When there is little energy available to digest and absorb food, a rotting process starts from within the food in much the same way as it would when you leave food items in the open for any length of time. The fermentation is responsible for the bloating, the distension of the abdomen, for constipation and/or diarrhoea. These rotten products—toxins—have to be dealt with by the system, which quickly makes them safe and 'stores' them. As there is an almost constant influx of toxins because of the continuing low inner energy, the accumulation grows larger almost by the day, resulting in major stress on the system, which eventually will lead to a collapse when it is no longer able to cope with the workload.

Effective treatment, as well as prevention, has to concentrate on the increase of inner energy and digestive fire. No treatment can be effective without it. Ear candling as a treatment has proven itself time and again as a very efficient method of increasing the quantity and quality of 'inner energy'.

Ear Candling

How can sticking a hollow candle in your ear and burning it do you any good at all? The crucial factor is the heat that is generated by the flame. There is no direct heat exchange between the candle and the body (the ear) of the person as the bottom of the candle never even gets warm. Yet the heat on the top of the candle is just as important as the heat in the open fire burning in the winter. You do not need to sit in the flames in order to absorb and benefit from the heat produced by the flames. The reason for this is radiation; the air around the fire warms up and transports that heat to the air which is in contact with your body. As the air immediately surrounding you warms up you become warm and feel cosy.

In a similar way, the fire on top of the candle heats the air *inside* the hollow candle. This creates a movement of air as the top part of the air column is much warmer than the lower regions. The warmer air starts to spiral downwards towards the bottom of the candle (observed by anybody who has ever done ear candling), taking with it the energy from the fire rather than just the warmth from the air. In the example of the open winter fire, the air moves linear from the fire to your body and creates a direct heat transfer. In ear candling the air moves spirally, whereby the air molecules in that particular motion transfer the heat (temperature, kinetic energy) from the top into an ever-increasing vortical movement, which cools the air but highly charges it. So, the temperature of the air moving quickly down inside the candle is cool but the energy is high. As this air now comes close to the layer of air-body contact, it releases that energy into the body. It is this energy input which will make all the difference to the state of health of the body.

Yet another view of how ear candling transfers healing energy to the human body is to draw a parallel with the ancient Chinese practice of moxibustion, which is a type of treatment performed by acupuncturists to stimulate energy into systems of deficiency, creating an improved level of health function in the corresponding area. The herb mugwort is compressed into a finger thick cylinder shape, of which one end is set on fire. This end is held either proximal to the area requiring stimulation or over an acupuncture point relating to the area. Ear candling is equally about having a flame, which creates and transfers energy, close to an area and acupuncture points relating to areas in need of healing. The region in which the ear candle is burning (the ear) is a complete acupuncture-point diagram of the entire body in the shape of an upside down foetus. One could easily conclude that there would be a marvellous influx of energy into the whole of the acupuncture meridian system.

Methods of Studying the Effects of Ear Candling

The authors have used various methods of research to obtain a clearer understanding of which systems are affected by ear candling and to what extent. The primary methods are active observation of clinic results and improvements in a variety of health conditions: kinesiology muscle testing (Touch for Health) and live blood cell analysis.

Live blood cell analysis is a marvellous tool to use in regard to treatment studies. It clearly shows in an almost snapshot manner the state of health of our being, as well as revealing health tendencies a person has experienced through various periods of life. One observes under very high magnification the blood and its constituents on a live one blood cell-thick layer preparation. The health of our blood cells, the presence of foreign pathogens, and the activity level of the cells, in particular the immune cells, can be directly evaluated. The cells of the immune system become much more active following ear candling treatment. They seem more able to sense the presence of foreign toxic material, move towards it with much greater speed and accuracy, and engulf the material with much greater ease. This fascinating direct observation helps to confirm why so many people note a rapid improvement after ear candling.

These visual findings have been confirmed in more detail through muscle testing. Kinesiology muscle testing is utilized by health professionals all over the world. The application of muscle testing is done by the practitioner pressing on the client's limb to ascertain if that particular muscle holds steady (locked) or lets go (unlocked). As every cell and every part of the body holds all information about everything that the system has ever experienced, the muscle will also have this 'database' at its disposal. The scope of information gained through muscle testing is only limited by the knowledge and skills of the practitioner and the desire to unearth true answers. It is thus that kinesiology confirms that not only the function of the white blood cells has become more precise and effective, but also that other aspects of the immune system have improved tremendously. The activity of all lymphocytes, phagocytes, T-cells, and B-cells is more targeted and direct, as well as bringing about improvements in the function of the spleen and thymus glands.

Effect on Body Systems

We all know that it is crucial in cancer treatment to maximize the immune system's potential. By destroying or inhibiting the function of the body's natural fighting mechanism we will leave the body weak and vulnerable, unable to defend itself. If ear candling is going to be of any use at all in cancer treatment it will at least have to provide support for the immune system, as indeed all cancer treatments should—unless you are not particularly bothered about the effect of the treatment on the whole patient.

Visual findings of improvement in immune function have been confirmed in more detail through muscle testing (kinesiology). Not only has the activity of the white blood cells become more precise and effective, other aspects of the immune system have also improved tremendously. The overall effect is that the whole of the immune system is more alert, more mobile, and more assertive after each ear candling session.

Lymphatic drainage, which apart from being an essential tool in the clearing out of toxic material also houses a vast array of immune cells, improves significantly with ear candling. Dramatic visual descriptions of swollen lymph glands disappearing under ear candling treatment, as snowballs in the sun, have been reported. More commonly, diffuse lymphatic swelling in the neck and throat area has been seen to disappear after treatment. Even finger swelling has diminished, as reported by individuals because of loosening of rings they wear.

The initial drainage is most notably seen in the area from the ears upwards, including the cranial cavity, sinuses, the area around the eyes, the middle and inner ear areas. This also establishes an unblocking of the cranial sutures (blockage of these causes a lot of problems as demonstrated in cranial osteopathy), a re-establishment of the articulation of the cranial sutures and of the smoothness in rhythm of the cerebral spinal fluid pumping mechanism, as well as the craniosacral articulation pump (again, such problems are highlighted in osteopathy). Further sessions drain the lymphatic system from the collarbone up; from the mid-chest up; from mid-abdomen up; down to the thighs, working its way towards the toes until the entire body's lymphatic system becomes really clear and functioning. Not only does this indicate the role ear candling plays in the cleansing of the body but it also shows the accumulative effect of regular ear candling sessions whereby the cleansing of tissues continues down the body structure, rather than having to start from scratch each time when we allow too much time to lapse between sessions.

A commonly recommended treatment schedule is 3 treatments of 2–4 candles per ear within 10 days. Three additional treatments of 2–4 ear candles per ear over the next 3–4 weeks. The number of candles per ear depends upon body size and level of congestion/ illness. The bigger and sicker a person is, the more they will benefit from additional candles in each treatment. After this six-treatment protocol, re-evaluate and proceed as required, aiming for 3–4 bursts of two sessions back-to-back per year. This will build a very strong level of health within the person on many levels.

With almost absolute predictability, the healing energy delivered to the body by the ear candling process will be delivered to the systems most in need. The body is a completely conscious being, knowing precisely what is happening with every cellular structure at all times. It will therefore provide the largest amount of corrective power to the systems in greatest need, a balancing effect to the areas less in need, bringing virtually all systems to an even platform of function, then raising the capacity of function across the board up to an optimal health level. In other words, what is most urgent will get the extra energy input first, and sometimes it isn't at all where we would have expected it.

Emotional Effect

Research in the last two decades has been able to demonstrate not only the fact that emotions influence our state of health but also that all feelings and emotions are translated into chemicals in all systems within the body. When people are in a stressful state their bodies biochemically produce stress-related chemicals. These chemicals have health-reducing effects such as: the stomach produces more acid and the duodenum more digestive juices in an erratic way; the mobility of the stomach and gut increases dramatically; circulation is constantly kept high; breathing becomes much more rapid and shallow. This serves to reduce the digestive fire for the burning of the food we consume, leading to a toxic build-up. The senses are heightened; the adrenals show a massive increase in activity; muscles are in a state of permanent tension, and so on. Stress also changes the blood flow patterns in the brain, in the limbic and endocrine systems draining blood away from those centres most responsible for clear, cognitive, emotionally balanced states of living.

Both states, stressed and relaxed, result in neuro-chemical activity: one producing highly toxic substances, the other very powerful healing chemicals. We have the ability to choose through our thoughts and actions the state we live in, stressed or relaxed. *We do have the choice!*

When a person is joyful, calm, peaceful, in a loving-centred state, that state of mind produces positive healing chemicals. Parts of the endocrine system, which are more active in a relaxed calm state, will be primarily: the pineal gland, the pituitary gland, the thalamus, and the hypothalamus. The amygdala and hippocampus (two parts of our limbic system controlling primal behaviours which monitor the presence of danger and sensory information, as well as mood control) will command less control in a relaxed, calm state.

Chemicals, produced as a direct result of our emotions, are responsible for how we physically feel. It is the long-term direction which these chemicals give to the tissues they govern that will produce either a long, well-balanced, non-stressful cell life or a disrupted, unbalanced, damage-inducing life. Cancer is certainly one of many eventual outcomes of a long-standing stressful and unbalanced cell stimulation or suppression.

A well-documented and universally agreed effect of ear candling is a feeling of complete relaxation. People always comment on how they could 'go to sleep' even during the treatment. This state produces the appropriate chemicals to reverse any negative and stress-induced effects under which the body may have been living for a considerable time; in other words, a *healing state*. The overall benefit on the health of the person in view of the above is now obvious.

In W. A Chapman's book *Your Cosmic Destiny* (Vantage Press, 1985), he describes experiments in the psychology laboratory that found hatred, anger, and jealousy caused different-coloured condensates from calmness and contentment, which upon analysis contained deadly poisons. The poison of a few minutes jealousy is enough to kill a guinea pig. An hour of hatred produces enough poison to kill 80 guinea pigs; on the other hand, happy, loving peaceful emotions produce some of the most powerful healing chemicals known to mankind.

If you have somebody who is in a cancer therapy treatment protocol, the thing which causes cancer to grow faster than anything else is fear. If a person is fearful, there is an automatic fight/flight state, which is prolonged for the whole time the fear resides within. The adrenals as well as the amygdala and hippocampus will be kicked into a very high functional level and the chemicals produced in the body as a consequence will be of a very toxic nature. Ear candling will instantaneously normalize the level of over-excitement in the function of these glands while dramatically boosting the systems that are in a low energy state—the pineal, the pituitary, the thalamus, the hypothalamus—systems responsible for producing very powerful healing neuro-chemicals. Ear candling has an instant effect on the entire glandular system and brain region energy distribution in a very positive manner. Within the space of a few treatments ear candling works to bring the entire glandular and limbic system to a very harmonious, ideal state of function. This is commonly achieved by the sixth session. As a result, people are more emotionally balanced; they are more enabled, feel more capable, relaxed, less threatened, and have more hope. Hope is a powerful 'molecule'.

The Life Force and Healing

The energy systems of our being—aura, chakras, and meridians—interface with our body's electrical system, the nervous system. The intertwined function of this group provides the electrical grid that delivers life force energy to *all parts* of our being, to each cell of our body. If the energy grid experiences disrupted flow, then a direct result will be a reduction or a disturbance to the function of the particular physical part supplied with this 'less than optimal energy'. This will directly reduce the health capacity of that part of the body. On the other hand, strengthening the energy systems provides us with excellent resistance to ill health.

In Chinese medicine the key factor to health is a strong balanced acupuncture meridian flow carrying *chi* 'life force' to all body parts. In particular, the kidney organ/meridian *yin* energy is seen as a vital store-house of life energy. Strengthening the state of kidney energy and its distribution is essential to any form of healing process. Clinical research has shown that, of the systems receiving healing energy from ear candling, the *yin* aspect of the kidney meridian is very often in the top three. This whole concept is of extreme importance to our health, and it is no surprise that in Chinese medicine the ears relate directly to the kidneys. Cold is damaging to the kidneys. With ear candling, the heat of the flame creates a reverse flush of energy back down to the kidneys filling them with warmth and vitality, providing a storehouse of 'life energy'.

In Indian medicine, it is the flow of *prana* 'life force' which determines the capacity for vitality in all body parts and aspects of our lives. The central part of the *prana* movement, the 'spine' as it were, is from the base of the physical spine upwards, coiled in a kind of double helix fashion around a central straight channel. The chakra at the base of the spine, called the root chakra, houses the 'life energy' and therefore has a very close connection with the physical body. It provides it with vitality and strength, and relates to our survival instinct and procreation. The root chakra has been shown to react very quickly and positively to ear candling, gaining power and strength. From here, more energy will be distributed all the way up the spine fanning out into all body tissues. The upward movement of this energy, our life force, travels into the brain region, stimulates key areas, and then opens and strengthens the crown chakra. This chakra—the place of the fontanel (the soft spot on a baby's head)—provides us with access to the universal healing energy (*yang* energy).

We find evidence of this in clinical research showing the posterior aspect of the pituitary gland (a *yin* consciousness-building centre) to be the system with the highest priority for receiving healing energy from ear candling. Clients often develop greater inward strength and self-knowledge from continued applications of ear candling (*yin* consciousness), often translated into less fear and greater personal assurance.

The free flow of 'life energy' is enhanced as a result of ear candling, clearing, and strengthening all aspects of the chakras, meridians, and aura. Hence the entire energy grid is much improved in its ability to deliver life force energy to every cell in our body. Cells in a state of poor health will rely on the powerful input of this life force energy to be able to regain health.

Conclusion

As shown, illness is created by long-standing stress on the natural processes. The cumulative effect of this situation leads to physical malfunctioning, such as cancer. As the only things that caused the disease are the body and the mind, so they are the only things that can ever heal it. The healing will have to come from inside, and can only be achieved by supporting and sustaining a natural balance within the functions of the whole body-mind person.

In order to relieve the stress caused by progressive malfunctioning, one has to clean up the system as best as one can. This can be achieved through stimulation and support of the elimination systems. To this effect, it is essential to reduce the negative influences and build-up of toxins, to strengthen the immune system, and to increase elimination. All these processes require extra energy input. Ear candling not only delivers that extra energy, it also mobilizes the immune system throughout; it increases lymphatic drainage allowing areas to be cleaned up; and it delivers through positive mood changes a series of balancing chemicals which bring the whole systemic function back into smooth operation, creating an environment conducive to healing and the building of health.

· · ·

PATRICK QUANTEN, MD, works as a teacher and therapist and has developed his own techniques of bodywork, using only natural healing methods and traditional skills, which consist of stimulating the body's healing system. More information on ear candling and on his work in general can be found on his website: *http://freespace.virgin. net/ahcare.qua/index.html.*

GREG WEBB, RMT, lives and works in Calgary, Canada, teaching Touch for Health and ear candling. He makes his own candles, which he uses for a variety of pathologies, and he has a very deep understanding of kinesiology and its application to enhance the communication system with the body. He can be contacted through his website: *www.gregwebb.ca.*

CHAPTER 6

Echoes from the International Ear Candling Conference

The International Ear Candling Conference was held in 2006 and provided an excellent opportunity to learn about what else candling can do.

One of the participating candle therapists told me that she had been consulted by a patient who announced that she had a perforated ear drum. The therapist agreed to see her, but discovered there was a much larger hole in the eardrum than she had imagined. She told the patient she should consult her GP before receiving a treatment. The lady explained that she had suffered from a massive infection in a Eustachian tube and went periodically to the hospital where a drain was put through the hole into the Eustachian tube to draw out the infected fluid. She understandably found the procedure excruciating. Greatly reassured that she couldn't do more harm than that with a candle, the therapist agreed to proceed. After one treatment the patient felt huge relief, and after the second visit a week later the infection had completely cleared up.

The second story from the same therapist concerned a lady whom she treated with four pairs of ear candles in a single session, and yet was still asking for more. This is where consulting a competent therapist is very important and this therapist was sufficiently experienced to know that the patient had had enough. Following the session, while the lady was walking down the street, an HGV pulled up with a whoosh of its airbrakes, and she reported later that she found the sound almost unbearable; any more treatments that day and loud noises would have caused her real pain.

People have often asked if ear candles are suitable for animals, and this therapist confirmed that a friend with a long-eared dog holds a candle in place, wrapping his ear round it. The dog loves the treatment and, when she gets the candles out and the he can smell the ingredients, he rushes up to see if they might be for him.

Someone else I know told me that her very trusting cat, a frequent sufferer from canker, allowed her to use a quarter of a candle in each ear. Her husband holds the cat, wrapped gently in a cloth, during the treatment, which has proved very successful.

One very experienced therapist told of a patient with only one ear. She treated the ear that was present and for the other side, she took a candle and sealed up the end so that no smoke would emanate from the bottom. She held it just over the place where the entrance to the auditory canal would have been. The patient thanked her afterwards by saying that he felt very balanced. As has been pointed out elsewhere, because the warmth and the energy of the flame spiral down the candle, closing the end in no way detracts from the treatment. You do not even need to close the end; this is only so that greasy residue doesn't get deposited on the patient's skin.

Closing the candle at the bottom can overcome many problems and the patient is still benefiting from the energy of the warmth and the flame. In fact, a therapist I have trained told me that he systematically closes the end of the candle before all his treatments. It also answers all those naysayers who insist that the action of the candle damaged the ear irretrievably.

Canadian therapist Greg Webb, whose paper written in collaboration with Dr Patrick Quanten constitutes Chapter 5, was applying ear candles to someone who had taken antibiotics six months earlier for an ear infection. There was a large plug of old wax that needed to come out, and it is his practice to clean the area round the entrance to the auditory canal with cotton buds dipped in hydrogen peroxide afterwards (a procedure mentioned earlier). When the solution bubbles, it indicates there is still some infection present in the ear. He needed to use several cotton buds on the infection which, in his opinion, had been stabilized but not eliminated by antibiotics.

Webb cited another case of a man who had worn hearing aids for over 40 years and who was able to hear quite well with them. He received around 20 treatments over a six-month period, with a total of over 20 candles per ear, and can now hear better without his hearing aids than he could before with them in place. His wife, diagnosed with progressive nerve deterioration by her doctor, also found her hearing ability improved when she received ear candle treatments. Compared with the cases presented in earlier chapters, this does go to prove that we all have different needs, and what works rapidly for some requires far more time for others.

Webb told conference attendees that one of the most exciting candling success stories he had heard had been related to him by another practitioner. A man of 93, blind for several years as a result of glaucoma, was treated for a whole afternoon with 7–8 candles per ear. As he was being driven home, he could see the white line in the middle of the road, and when he arrived he was able to see his wife's face for the first time in several years. (See Chapter 2: Glaucoma.)

Body Candling

Body candling is exactly as the name implies: candling elsewhere on the body rather than just the ears. It opens up a whole new field of application for the candles. I discovered it several years ago and have seen some amazing results. My professional students love it, and they, too, have found it to be extremely effective.

The lymphatic drainage provided just by using the candles in the ears can be felt throughout the body (see Chapter 5), and there have been reports of swollen lymph glands relaxing and even fingers, where rings were embedded, have returned to their normal size. Body candling can, indeed, offer a plus, targeted at the area that most needs the energy.

The patient remains fully clothed on the treatment table while a candle is placed on something like a paper tissue over the area to be treated. The energy from the warmth of the candle will then penetrate rapidly to the root of the problem. It has been found that a candle over the navel (the source of life) is very pleasant and can be used for stubborn constipation. I also had a good result with this method on a patient suffering from a spastic colon.

A therapist who contacted me about body candling explained that a friend of hers had wanted to become pregnant but was resisting the physical changes this would bring to her body. She candled her in her navel and in a very short time the friend was pregnant. So what had changed? Impossible to say and perhaps she would have conceived anyway, but I offer the information as another example where, although we have no direct proof, it can add to our knowledge of body candling. My fact sheet on women and candles (which can be downloaded from my website) gives more information on using a candle in the navel, why, and what the consequences may be. It also explains the use of candling post-partum. This relates to many Eastern traditions of treating women who have just delivered a child or who have had a miscarriage.

A candle in the navel has also been found to be extremely effective for treating digestive problems, poor peristalsis, male and female sexual disorders, even as part of a slimming diet. However, I would add a note of caution here: care *must* be taken when candling the navel as, for example, it can open the door to memories of past sexual abuse or a condition that the therapist has little experience in managing. I never normally recommend it unless I know the person well.

To give an example, on my professional courses I always give students the opportunity of using a candle elsewhere on the body after candling the ears. One student, with many therapies to her credit and who was studying intestinal massage at the same time, opted for a candle in the navel. Fortunately, we were at the end of the day as, a short while afterwards, she was overcome with feelings of nausea and had to walk home in the fresh air to clear her head. I spoke to her the next day and she was fine, but if someone with experience of working on the intestines has such a strong reaction, it pays to be very prudent with this area of the body.

Canadian therapist Greg Webb has experimented widely with body candling and uses kinesiology to decide where on the body he should burn a candle; it is not always the most obvious place. He has found that when the patient has had his/her ears candled earlier, the treatment is more effective. One of the conditions for which he has frequently used body candling is during a woman's monthly cycle, when breast congestion can occur. He starts with a candle between the breasts to drain the lymph and then uses one or more candles over any particular lymph node(s) that feel(s) tender (this is mentioned in my fact sheet). Candling between the breasts is also recommended for a new mother who has difficulty in producing milk.

As is the case in moxibustion (which has a similar effect), body candling can be done over meridian points. Because these lines crisscross the body, there are many that pass in proximity to the ears. One

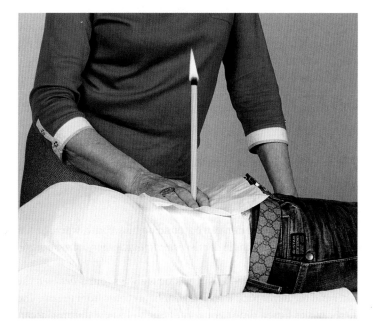

thing is certain: as with ear candling, body candling can do no harm and has been seen to produce some wonderful results.

A good illustration of body candling and the benefit of regular treatments occurred in a patient who came to me every month. One day she arrived with the feeling of a tight band across her forehead. I treated her ears and offered to burn a half candle over the space between and just above her eyes (the third-eye chakra). As she was leaving, she said she felt lighter and her headache had gone. The following month she told me that after the treatment some hard crusty stuff had come out of her nose. We both realized that because she was candled regularly something had shifted and this was the result. I'm not saying that if she had been a first-time patient the same would not have happened, but it is less likely.

One of the differences of opinion in candling has been on the debris found in the candles. When they are used purely for ears, many people—including me in the early days—swore it was ear wax mixed with candle residue. Dr Patrick Quanten, who with Greg Webb contributed Chapter 5 on candling and cancer, insists that it is purely an indication of the state of the body. Here is a brief summary of his comments:

> The debris never comes out of the body. It is an expression of the energetic changes that have happened in the human energy field. The powder is an expression of the amount of water that has been 'dried out', and the amount of fat that appears indicates the amount of energy the system has stored, has taken up from the candle. Ear candling is an energetic thing, not a physical one.

More detailed information can be found on his website, where he has posted an article on candle debris: *http://freespace.virgin.net/ahcare.qua/index.html.*

As mentioned earlier, as the residue is always found *between* the filter and the burnt part, it is obvious it hasn't come from the ear. The first candles I used didn't contain filters, so I knew nothing about that then.

One therapist I trained, who very often uses body candling combined with other therapies, has also proved Quanten's point. She opens the candle stub after a treatment and often finds the same little brown lumps that can appear after candling the ear. Sometimes, as when treating the ears, she finds nothing at all, the contents of each candle providing information on the energy level of the patient.

Although ear candling in itself is extremely powerful and works to put the body into a relaxed state—just listen to the gurgling of a patient's intestine when it is being done—burning a candle over the area that is causing pain or discomfort works even faster. Remember: always candle the ears first, unless they have recently been treated, as this will lead to a better result.

Candle Courses

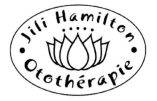

With the increase in popularity of complementary therapies worldwide, there has been an on-going drive in recent years toward professional accreditation of individual therapies, whereby students receive specialized training from certified instructors, carry out case studies, and are then awarded diplomas upon successful completion of the required number of hours of coursework. Ear candling (or ototherapy, as it is known in Switzerland) is no different in this respect. As therapists, it is in our interest to reassure our patients that we have studied and understood ototherapy and its vast field of application, so that we can answer questions and treat the many different pathologies and health conditions that we are likely to encounter in professional practice in a skilled and ethical way designed to ensure the highest level of success.

I regularly organize courses in ototherapy for therapists who work with a body therapy such as massage, reflexology, or an energy therapy such as Reiki or crystals. These courses, which are also open to trainee therapists, are recognized in Switzerland by the Fondation suisse pour les médecines complémentaires (ASCA), the main professional body, and patients consulting practitioners trained by me and holding complementary medical insurance can be reimbursed by certain companies. The normal civil responsibility insurance, to which all practitioners in Switzerland are required to subscribe, covers candle treatments as well.

Courses are held throughout the year, generally at my home in Geneva, but I am prepared to travel anywhere in Switzerland, France or Belgium. Should anyone wish to set up a course, I will be delighted to come and teach it. If you're looking to participate in a course in your area, please contact me as I often have a list of people waiting for a suitable date or a course nearer to where they live.

As I am fluent in both English and French, participants may request courses and/or course materials in either language.

I also offer mini courses to non-therapists who want to know more about the candles, what they do, the contraindications and the correct manner in which to give a treatment to family and friends. For further details, see my website (*www.jilihamilton.com*) or e-mail me at *info@jilihamilton.com*.

NOTE: Professional courses are held in many countries. It is important to check which of these are covered by professional insurance and which are recognized by any professional body to which you may belong, as requirements vary greatly from country to country. I have no information as to legal requirements and courses available in the US, and they probably vary from state to state. In Switzerland, for example, although certificates of competence are recognized country-wide, the requirements with which each practitioner has to comply vary widely from canton to canton.

Courses include those organized by Greg Webb, RMT in Canada *(http://gregwebb.ca)*; in the UK by Dr Patrick Quanten *(http://freespace.virgin.net/ahcare.qua/index.html)*; also in the UK by Mary Dalgleish and Lesley Hart *(www.head2toemassage.co.uk)*, and by Sue Maunsell and Linda Stokes. Sue and Linda's course is known as Thermo-Auricular Therapy®. They train therapists from many other countries, but it is the responsibility of individual therapists to check with the relevant licensing authorities in their home countries about what they need to do to be recognized as certified candle practitioners.

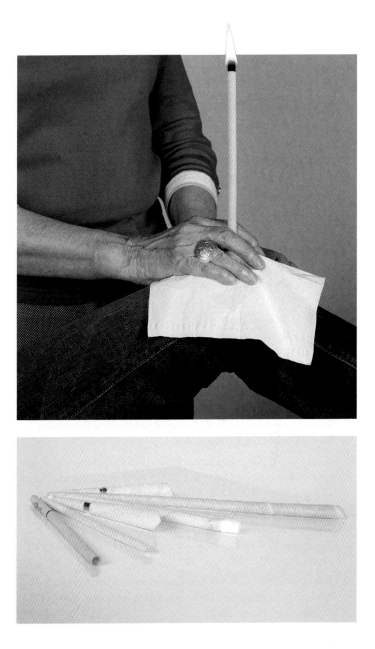

Notes

1. J. Durga, P. Verhof, et al. 'Effects of Folic Acid Supplementation on Hearing in Older Adults – A Randomized Control Trial', 2007.

2. T. Dunder, L.Kuikka, et al. 'Diet, Serum Fatty Acids and Atopic Diseases in Childhood', *Allergy*, 2001, 56, 5.

3. Sanchez, A., et al. 'Role of Sugars in Human Neutrophilic Phagocytosis', *American Journal of Clinical Nutrition*. Nov 1973; 261:1180_1184.

4. Bernstein, J., et al. 'Depression of Lymphocyte Transformation Following Oral Glucose Ingestion', *American Journal of Clinical Nutrition*.1997;30:613.

5. Uhari, M., Kontiokari, T., et al. 'Xylitol Chewing Gum in Prevention of Acute Otitis Media, Double Blind Randomised Trial', *British Medical Journal* 313, 1996.

6. Spiro, D.M., et al. 'Otitis Media, A Randomized Controlled Trial', 2006.

7. Tien, D.C., Tseng, K.H., et al. 'Colloidal Silver Fabrication Using the Spark Discharge System and Its Antimicrobial Effect on *Staphylococcus aureus*', Graduate Institute of Mechanical and Electrical Engineering, Da-An District, Taipei, 2008.

8. Kaur, M., et al. 'Grapeseed Extract Induces Cell Cycle Arrest and Apoptosis in Human Colon Carcinoma Cells', University of Colorado Cancer Center, Denver, USA, 2008.

9. Jolly, Rajan Singh. 'The Twelve Cell Salts of Schüssler and Their Role in Maintaining Health', 2012 *(http://ezinearticles.com/? The-Twelve-Cell-Salts-Of-Schussler-And-Their-Use-For-Maintaining-Health&id=6834540)*.

10. Ivory, et al. 'Oral Delivery of Lactobacillus *casei Shirota* Modifies Allergen-Induced Immune Responses in Allergic Rhinitis'. *Clinical & Experimental Allergy*, 2008.

11. Mukhopadhyay, C., Basak, C., et al. 'A Comparative Analysis of Bacterial Growth with Earphone Use', Department of Microbiology, Kasturba Medical College, 2008.

12. Rabinowitz, P.M. 'Hearing Loss and Personal Music Players', *BMJ*, April, 2010.

13. Johnson, E.S., Kadam, N.P., Hylands, D.M., et al. 'Efficacy of Feverfew as Prophylactic Treatment of Migraine', *Br Med J (Clin Res Ed.*), 1985.

14. Diener, H.C., Pfaffenrath, V., et al. 'Efficacy and Safety of 6.25 mg t.i.d. Feverfew CO2-extract (MIG-98) in Migraine Prevention— a Randomized, Double-Blind, Multicentre, Placebo-Controlled Study', 2006.

15. Bigal, M.R., Kurth, T., Santello, N., et al. 'Migraine and Cardiovascular Disease', 2010.

16. Hutter, H.P., Moshammer, H., Wallner, P., et al. 'Tinnitus and Mobile Phone Use', Medical University of Vienna, 2010.

17. Morgenstern, C., Biermann, E. 'The Efficacy of Gingko Special Extract EGb 761 in Patients with Tinnitus', [translated from German], Allgemeines Krankenhaus St. Georg, Hamburg, 2002.

18. *http://umm.edu/health/medical/altmed/herb/ginkgo-biloba.*

19. Deoni, S.C., Dean, D.C. 3rd., Piryatinsky I., et al., 'Breastfeeding and Early White Matter Development: A Cross-Sectional Study', Advanced Baby Imaging Lab, School of Engineering, Brown University, Providence, USA, 2013.

20. Kang D. -W., Park J.G., et al. 'Reduced Incidence of *Prevotella* and Other Fermenters in Intestinal Microflora of Autistic Children', 2013.

21. *http://www.youtube.com/watch?v=3wwDPcNdxJQ 2*

22. Klein, N.P., Bartlett, J., et al. 'Waning Protection After Fifth Dose of Acellular Pertussis Vaccine in Children', Kaiser Permanente, 2012.

23. Curhan, S.C., Eavey, R., et al. 'Analgesic Use and the Risk of Hearing Loss in Men', 2010.

Bibliography

Abehsera, Michel. *The Healing Power of Clay: Natural Remedy for Dozens of Common Ailments*. New York, USA: Citadel Press/Kensington Books, 2001.

Abehsera, Michel. *The Healing Clay*, 1987 (out of print).

Adams, Zoe. *The Colloidal Silver Report*. Germany: Another Country Publishing, 2003 (out of print).

Berthoud, Françoise Dr. *Mon enfant, a-t-Il besoin d'un pédiatre?* Switzerland: Editions Ambre, 2006.

Buchman, Dian Dincin (Ph.D). *The Complete Book of Water Healing: Using Earth's Most Essential Resource to Cure Illness, Promote Health, and Soothe and Restore Body, Mind, and Spirit.* Second edition. New York, USA: McGraw Hill, 2001.

Chapman, W. A. *Your Cosmic Destiny*. New York, USA: Vantage Press, 1958 (out of print).

Clark, Susan. *What Really Works in Natural Health?* London, UK: Bantam, 2004.

Coleman, Vernon, Dr. *Food for Thought: Your Guide to Healthy Eating.* Second revised edition. London, UK: The European Medical Journal Publishing House, 2000.

Courtney, Hazel. *What's the Alternative?* Second edition. London, UK: Boxtree Ltd/MacMillan, 1996.

Dalgleish, Mary and Lesley Hart. *Ear Candling: The Essential Guide.* CreateSpace Independent Publishing Platform, 2013.

de Vries, Jan. *Healing in the 21ˢᵗ Century : Complementary Medicine and Modern Life*. Edinburgh, UK: Mainstream Publishing, 2005.

Dethlefsen, Thorwald and Dr Rüdiger Dahlke. *The Healing Power of Illness: The Meaning of Symptoms and How to Interpret Them*. Shaftsbury, Dorset, UK: Element Books, 1997 (English edition).

Dextreit, Raymond. *Our Earth, Our Cure*. New York, USA: Citadel Press/ Kensington Books, 1987 reissue.

Geiger, Gisela Elisabeth. *Les sels minéraux de Schüssler: Manuel pour se guérir soi-même*. France: Ed Trédaniel, 2002 (translated from German).

Holford, Patrick, BSC DipION FBANT NTCRP, and Dr James Braly. *Hidden Food Allergies : Is What You Eat Making You Ill?* London, UK: Piatkus/Little Brown, 2006.

Knishinsky, Ran. *The Clay Cure: Natural Healing from the Earth.* Rochester, VT, USA: Healing Arts Press/Inner Traditions/Bear and Company, 1998.

Page, Christine R. Dr., *The Mirror of Existence: Stepping into Wholeness*. London, UK: C.W. Daniel, 1995.

Perrin, F.G., *La correction de l'atlas: Découverte fondamentale ou supercherie?* Switzerland: Ed. à la Carte, 2006.

Pert, Candace. *Molecules of Emotion*: *Why you Feel the Way you Feel*. New York, USA: Hay House, 1997.

Roberts, H.J. *Aspartame Disease: An Ignored Epidemic*, USA: Sunshine Sentinel Press, Inc., 2001.

Sceats, Andrew. *Ear Candling and Other Treatments for Ear, Nose and Throat Problems*. Shrewsbury, UK: Pressuredown Therapies, 2010.

Smith, Jeffrey, M. *Seeds of Deception*: *Exposing Corporate and Government Lies About the Safety of Genetically Engineered Food,* USA: Yes! Books, 2003.

Wagner, Dr Edward M. and Sylvia Goldfarb. *How to Stay Out of the Doctor's Office: An Encyclopedia for Alternative Healing*: Instant Improvement, Inc, New York, USA, 1994.

Weil, Andrew, Dr. *Spontaneous Healing: How to Discover and Embrace Your Body's Natural Ability to Maintain and Heal Itself*. New York, USA: Ballantine, 2000.

Welch, Robyn Elizabeth. *Conversations with the Body: The True Sixth Sense Story of a Medical Intuitive*. London, UK: Hodder & Stoughton, 2002.

White, Arthur, N.D., D.O. *Tinnitus*. The New Self-Help Series. London, UK: Thorsons, 1986.

Websites

- *www.netdoctor.co.uk*
- *www.naturalnews.com*
- *www.feingold.org*
- *www.wddty.com*
- *www.mpwhi.com*
- *www.preventdisease.com*
- *www.vernoncoleman.com*
- *www.medline.com*
- *www.healthwyze.org*
- *http://www.americanrevolution.org/medicine.html*
- *www.atlasprofilax.com*
- *http://freespace.virgin.net/ahcare.qua/index.html*
- *www.gregwebb.ca*
- *www.head2toemassage.co.uk*

Permissions

The quotation from *Molecules of Emotion* by Candace B. Pert Ph.D (with an Introduction by Deepak Chopra) is by kind permission of Simon & Schuster UK Limited, London.

About the Author

Jili Hamilton was born in England and has done a variety of jobs, including secretarial work, office administration, translating, bookselling, waitressing, and chamber-maiding. In 1987, she started studying reflexology with the Bayley School in Switzerland, obtaining a diploma in 1988. This opened her eyes to the world of complementary medicine, leading her to study many different therapies, including hands-on healing, Reiki, Indian head massage, metamorphic massage, lymphatic drainage, and so on. In 1991, she set up Hopi Products Limited in the UK, launching ear treatment candles on the British market at the Healing Arts Exhibition in London the same year. She has subsequently demonstrated and given talks on ear treatment candles at the major health exhibitions in England and Scotland, as well as participating in several radio and television programmes in Britain and in Switzerland. Some of the videos and articles are available to download on her website.

Jili now works as a teacher, therapist, and translator in Switzerland. She has also edited a book entitled *Messages from Beyond the Veil*, containing spirit writings by her grandmother, available from *www.amazon.co.uk*.

Her latest book, *A Seeker's Guide to a Life Worth Living*, published by O Books, came out in August 2013. Details are available on her website.

You may contact her by e-mail at *info@jilihamilton.com*, or visit her website at *www.jilihamilton.com*.

FINDHORN PRESS

Life-Changing Books

For a complete catalogue,
please contact:

Findhorn Press Ltd
117-121 High Street,
Forres IV36 1AB,
Scotland, UK

t +44 (0)1309 690582
f +44 (0)131 777 2711
e info@findhornpress.com

or consult our catalogue online
(with secure order facility) on
www.findhornpress.com

For information on the Findhorn Foundation:
www.findhorn.org